Nursing Beds
An Evaluation of the
effects of therapeutic
nursing

Nursing Beds
An evaluation
of the effects of
therapeutic nursing

Alan Pearson
PhD, MSc, RGN, ONC, RNT, DipN, FRCN

Sue Punton
RGN

Ismere Durant
MA Soc Sc

ROYAL COLLEGE OF NURSING
RESEARCH SERIES

Scutari Press

Aims of the Series
To encourage the appreciation and dissemination of nursing research by making relevant studies of high quality available to the profession at reasonable cost.

The RCN is happy to publish this series of research reports. The projects were chosen by the individual research worker and the findings are those of the researcher and relate to the particular subject in the situation in which it was studied. The RCN in accordance with its policy of promoting research awareness among members of the profession commends this series for study but views expressed do not necessarily reflect RCN policy.

Scutari Press

Viking House, 17–19 Peterborough Road,
Harrow, Middlesex HA1 2AX, England

A subsidiary of Scutari Projects, the publishing company of the Royal College of Nursing

British Library Cataloguing in Publication Data:
Pearson, Alan
    Nursing beds — an evaluation of the
    effects of therapeutic nursing.
    I. Title   II. Durant, Ismere   III. Punton, Sue
    610.73
    ISBN 1–871364–64–7

Typeset by Action Typesetting Limited, Gloucester
Printed and bound in Great Britain by
Billing & Sons Ltd, Worcester

Contents

Acknowledgements

Although all research involves many people other than the researchers, and the need to acknowledge this is common to all research endeavours, this study has been particularly reliant on a large number of people. This is largely so because of the nature of the study, and its political and philosophical ramifications.

Firstly, acknowledgement must be made to all of those who have worked in some way to enable the study to take place: the patients who agreed to participate; the staff of Oxford Nursing Development Unit; the staff of referring hospitals; the staff of the Radcliffe Infirmary, Oxford; and all who, in many ways, supported the clinical programme associated with the study. It is, of course, impossible to name everyone specifically and difficult to single out individuals. Mention must be made, however, of Liz Tutton and Richard McMahon (Nurse Practitioners), and Dr Ljuba Stirzaker, who accepted the day-to-day responsibility of providing therapeutic nursing to those who were admitted to the experimental nursing unit.

Secondly, members of the research team who painstakingly grappled with numerous data collection and retrieval problems, and who coped in circumstances not always associated with conducting a major study (such as inadequate office space and even more inadequate time availability). In this area, specific thanks are due to: Dr Adrian Smith and Dr Mark Starr, research assistants who analysed the data; Sue Bradshaw, who acted as external auditor; and the nursing units' ward co-ordinators who operated the randomisation centre and entered the raw data for computation. From Deakin University, we would like to thank Janine Sewart and Monika Loving for the typing, Susan Hocking for statistical assistance, and Miranda Hughes for her editorial assistance.

Thirdly, we are grateful to those who lent political and professional support to a project which evoked much scepticism and opposition to its belief in the value of nursing. Their constant support when things became difficult played a major part in mounting and continuing with the study. Their help could not have been done without. These supporters were numerous, but we particularly acknowledge the very real support of: Malcolm Ross, Dr Sean McCarthy, Dr Chris Paine, David Wilson, Shirley Williams and all the staff of Oxfordshire Health Authority Nursing Department.

Finally, though not least, we gratefully acknowledge the strong support of the Monument Trust and Hugh DeQueteville. This support has been both financial and conceptual. Through Mr DeQueteville, the Monument Trust has consistently expressed its understanding and support of the nature of nursing and of the beliefs which underlie the study. For this, we are both grateful and cognisant of its significance to the future development of nursing as a component of health care.

Alan Pearson (Geelong, Australia)
Sue Punton (Oxford)
Ismere Durant (Oxford)

1 Introduction to the study

This report is an account of a study into the effects of admitting people to an experimental unit based on therapeutic nursing, carried out in Oxfordshire from January 1986 to March 1987. This study was essentially a modified replication of a smaller study conducted in the same health district (Pearson et al, 1987) and both were funded by a research grant from the Monument Trust, with organisational support from Oxfordshire Health Authority. The underlying assumptions of both studies relate to the contemporary evolution of a clearer vision of the nursing role and the contribution that professional nursing can make to patients in hospital settings.

Prior to the emergence of 'modern' nursing, associated with the reforms instigated by Nightingale and her contemporaries, nursing was essentially an expressive activity, highly valued by sections of the community and distinctly different to medical intervention. The changes emanating from the modernisation of nursing towards the end of the 19th century included the linking of nursing with medical practice, and a subsequent belief that nursing was an adjunct to medicine, focusing largely on supporting the medical practitioner by becoming his 'eyes and ears', and administrator of his prescribed treatments. With the growth of medical science, and the associated move of health care from community bases to centralised hospitals, a plethora of specialised paramedical occupations developed.

The prevailing medical and lay ideology views patients with acute onset of illness (or in biological crisis) as being in need of medical assessment, diagnosis and treatment, and this is seen as best being provided in acute general hospitals. Resolution of the crisis is perceived to be the role of medical practitioners who apply

1

medical therapy and paramedical workers who apply specialist therapies. These 'therapists' are perceived to be instrumental in the resolution of biological crises, and thus their role and skill is referred to as therapeutic. Nursing is generally seen as a supporting activity, revolving around the so-called 'simple, basic' acts of daily living, essential in maintaining the integrity of the patient whilst the therapist engages in arresting or reversing the biological crisis. Nursing is therefore not usually perceived as a therapy, nor is it ascribed a therapeutic role.

This study arose from the growing belief in nursing that the provision of 'good' nursing is indeed therapeutic, and that nursing can make a difference to recovery and the overall outcomes of hospitalisation. Whilst the instrumental intervention of medical practitioners and paramedical therapists undoubtedly has a powerful effect on recovery, the provision of physical and psycho-social care, and health teaching are also seen as interventions which can have a powerful effect on patients. This latter form of professional intervention is legitimately a part of the nursing role and has, to date, been devalued in terms of its therapeutic effect.

Whilst initial admission to an acute unit, with a high level of medical and paramedical intervention, is usually essential for those in biological crisis, transfer to a unit where the caring, nurturing role of the nurse can predominate is seen as a useful strategy for the health care system.

Although nursing in any setting, including acute hospital wards, can be delivered in a therapeutic way, the pressures of time and technology frequently prevent nurses from focusing on their core caring and nurturing role, and the effects of it can be obscured. This study set out to establish a unit where an ideology of therapeutic nursing could prevail and where nursing could take the primary leadership role in planning patient care. The setting up and operations of this unit are described elsewhere but the philosophical underpinning of the unit was consistent with contemporary values expressed by nurses.

Currently, British nursing is advocating that the task-oriented approach of traditional nursing of the past needs to be abandoned in hospital care and an holistic, patient-centred approach is favoured. Nursing is characterised by rapid change and re-examination of fundamental values. Nursing care is becoming more systematic and concerned with the whole person;

conceptual analyses of the role of nursing have been developed, and are being applied as frameworks for assessment and intervention; and the previous, passive role of the patient is being questioned. All of these developments are said to constitute a reappraisal of the nursing role and to lead to a heightening of professional functioning. Accountability is developing, and managerial and organisational changes are taking place as a result. There is growing acceptance of 'primary nursing', where nurses accept responsibility and accountability for the care they give to a defined caseload.

Despite the apparent logic behind such moves, and anecdotal evidence to support the view that they have benefits both in cost effectiveness and quality care, there is too little objective evidence to confirm that nursing actually makes a difference and that contemporary trends give rise to 'better' nursing.

This study is an attempt to establish whether or not nursing is therapeutic and whether or not the new norms being advocated by nursing leaders enhance therapeutic effectiveness.

2 | Background to the study

THE PILOT AND THE PURPOSE

Oxfordshire Health Authority has, for some years, been committed to the development of clinical nursing and expansion of the nursing role. Therefore, in 1981, Burford, a small rural community hospital in Oxfordshire, was designated as a nursing development unit, the purpose being to explore and pilot new approaches to the practical delivery of nursing care.

Burford Hospital was a nine-bed unit with a traditional style of organising nursing care: nursing practice was task-oriented rather than professionally-oriented and nursing was based on a medical rather than a nursing model.

From 1981 to 1983 an intensive programme of staff development was introduced, both for nurses and members of the multi-disciplinary clinical team. Radical innovations were successfully introduced and it was established that the unit would primarily provide a professional 24 hour nursing service.

Primary nursing became well established, the nurse acting as key worker with 24 hour accountability for her patients. Practice was based on a **nursing** model with a clearly defined philosophy of nursing. Nurses worked in partnership with their patients – giving informed choice care which was patient-centred, rather than task-centred, and thereby individualised care for each patient became the 'norm'. The major pre- and post-change work norms at the Burford Hospital are represented in Figure 2.1.

These innovations in nursing at Burford were regularly written about in national nursing journals (Pearson, 1983, 1985; Swaffield, 1983). In one such article it was stated 'One idea is to use Burford to evaluate properly the different ways of managing care' (Swaffield, 1983).

PRE-CHANGE WORK NORMS	POST-CHANGE WORK NORMS
PATIENTS: Seen as old and dirty; not in need of professional nursing if not ill Patients liked routine. Patients passive.	Seen as individuals who need help to become independent and therefore in need of professional nursing, whether ill nor not. Patients liked having 'own nurse'. Patients liked freedom to choose own routine, be involved in care, read own notes.
NURSING CARE: Could be given by any worker, trained or untrained. Routinised and task centred. Directive and protective. Unplanned, based on judgemental criteria.	Given only by nurses. Flexible, individualised. Non-directive. Systematically planned, attempted to be objective.
DOCTORS: Unquestioned leaders. Admitted and discharged all patients.	Team work highly valued. Primary nurse seen as co-ordinator. Doctor's leadership questioned when patient's problems not primarily medical. Nurse co-ordinated team decisions to discharge. Nurse involved in decision to admit.
PHYSIOTHERAPIST: Gave all direct physiotherapy with little nursing involvement.	Physiotherapy taught to patient and nurse and incorporated into nursing plan.
OUTSIDE STAFF: All staff regarded as outsiders except nurses, auxiliaries and domestics.	All staff regarded as insiders except doctors.
OWNERSHIP OF PATIENTS: Patients 'owned' by doctors	Patients 'owned' by primary nurses.
NURSES: Goal = cure and getting through the work. Role = supervising untrained, operationalising doctor's orders. Accountable to doctor/nursing officer.	Goal = independent patients. Role = giving care. Accountable to patient and peer group.
NURSING OFFICER: Role = supervisor.	Role = consultant.

Figure 2.1 Pre- and post-change work norms at Burford Hospital

This idea was to become the pilot study, to test the belief that post-crisis patients could benefit from admission to the nursing unit, as opposed to staying in an acute unit. In acute illness, the patient is admitted to hospital for 24 hour medical care with nursing and support from other health workers: when the biological crisis of illness is resolved, the need for medical care falls and the patient's primary need is for rehabilitative care including nursing (Pearson, 1983). The need for nursing increases, but many hospital settings do not organise patient care in this way. The system is such that nurses would seem to concentrate on moving with the medical practitioners to the next patient in biological crisis. A nursing unit was required where patients could be transferred when the biological crisis was resolved and nursing would be the major therapy.

'Nursing beds – an alternative health care provision' (Pearson et al, 1987) is an unpublished report of the study to examine the feasibility and effects of establishing nursing beds in the British National Health Service (NHS), and compares the outcomes of patients admitted to the nursing unit with those who remained in acute wards.

The 2 year study conducted from 1983 to 1985 was funded by a generous grant awarded by the Monument Trust, enabling three further nursing beds to be situated within the nursing unit.

In a group of elderly people who had undergone internal fixation of a fractured neck of femur, the patient outcomes were compared between a control group remaining in the acute hospital and another group transferred from the acute hospital to Burford Nursing Development Unit, where nursing was advocated as the chief therapeutic activity.

The main objective was to attempt to establish whether the quality of nursing care in the nursing unit would be at least as good as that in the acute unit and whether or not the cost of nursing patients in the nursing unit would exceed the costs of nursing similar patients in other hospital wards.

Patients were referred for possible entry into the study by two consultant orthopaedic surgeons and informed consent was sought from the patients. Eighty two patients were allocated to control group (1), 25 were randomised to control group (2) and 45 were randomised to the nursing unit (3) (Figure 2.2).

All patients were interviewed on discharge, 6 weeks after discharge and 6 months after discharge, using a structured interview schedule (Appendix).

On discharge from hospital no significant differences were found between the groups in independence level, patients'

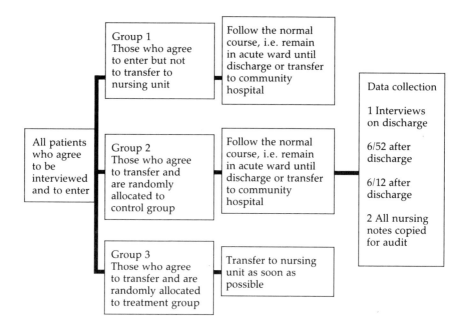

Figure 2.2 Nursing beds – an alternative health care provision.

expressed satisfaction with hospital care or in life satisfaction score. After 6 months, dependency had decreased for all groups with no significant difference between the groups. However, the amount of professional assistance needed by the patient at home in the 6 months following discharge was twice as much for the control patients as for those patients discharged from the nursing unit. Also at the 6 month interview, it was shown that life satisfaction had increased significantly for those patients admitted to the nursing unit.

Except for the quality of nursing received, the frequency of using stairs and the consultant responsible for medical care in the acute hospital, the three groups of patients did not differ significantly at the outset. However, the patients randomised to the nursing unit spent significantly less time in an acute hospital (with a median stay of only 7 days compared with 13 days for the patients randomised to the control group and 21 days for the patients who refused to be randomised at all). Thus, although the total length of hospital stays were the same, the nursing unit clearly fulfilled its objective of reducing the pressure on the acute hospital. The remaining question, therefore, is what effect did the nursing unit have on those patients who were randomised to it?

Although the three groups of patients did not differ significantly at the outset, during the following 6 months certain trends could be observed.

The degree of patient dependency decreased markedly during the 6 months following discharge, with the mean dependency scores for each group falling from about 25 to 20. This presumably represents an improvement in self-reliance caused by a recovery from the acute effects of the operation.

The Life Satisfaction Index (LSI) of patients in the three groups differed very significantly in both magnitude and direction in the 6 months following discharge.

The LSI of the patients who refused to be randomised declined steadily from a mean score of nearly 9 on discharge (the maximum score being 18) to (only) just over 6 at the third interview 6 months later. The LSI of patients who were randomised to the control group did not change significantly ($p = 0.37$) between the first and the third interviews, the score remaining about 8.5 thoughout the experiment. By contrast, the LSI of the patients admitted to the nursing unit increased significantly ($p = 0.02$) from a value of 9.6 at the outset to 11.0, some 6 months later. In view of the small numbers of patients involved in this trial, it is probably wiser not to overinterpret the LSI data, but it can at least be said that those patients randomised to the nursing unit were certainly no less happy than their counterparts randomised to the normal hospital ward.

The nursing audit scores showed that the quality of nursing differed very significantly between the groups. The quality of nursing was higher, and consistently so, in the nursing unit.

The quality of nursing was considerably better in the nursing unit ($p < 0.0001$). Indeed, not only was the mean nursing audit score for patients in the nursing unit some 50% higher than that of the control patients, but the variance of the nursing audit score was also much lower ($p < 0.001$). This indicated that the quality of nursing care for patients in the control group was not consistent and was prone to fluctuations with the audit scores ranging from 196 (excellent) to 55 (poor).

Considering this difference in nursing audit scores, it is surprising that the patients' opinions of the quality of nursing did not differ significantly between the two groups of randomised patients. This may be because elderly patients are easily satisfied, did not know what standard of care to expect or were afraid of the possibility of reprisals from the nursing staff if they were too critical.

Costings between the groups showed that nursing patients in the nursing unit incurred no more cost than those in acute beds. No significant difference was found between the group in total length of stay in NHS care, though patients randomised to the nursing unit spent significantly less time in acute beds.

The final unanswered question is whether the features that seem to characterise the nursing unit (i.e. length of stay in an acute hospital, the quality of nursing care and patient's life-satisfaction) are specific to the nursing unit or common to all community hospitals, of which the nursing unit is a specific case. Therefore, a second set of comparisons between the patients randomised to the nursing unit and community hospital was made. The results from this comparison must be treated with caution since patients were not randomised to a community hospital.

In brief, the results indicate that patients who were referred to the community hospitals tended to stay longer in an acute hospital (the median acute hospital stays were 11.5 days and 7.0 days); received poorer quality nursing ($p<0.0001$) but had a similar life satisfaction (LSI) score in comparison with patients randomised to the nursing unit. In the 6 weeks following discharge, patients in the two randomised groups received approximately the same amount of professional assistance. However, between the second and third interview (6 weeks and 6 months) after discharge, patients randomised to the control group received more than twice as many visits from the professional services per patient than those randomised to the nursing unit. The bulk of these extra visits were from the home help services, who visited about a third of patients in the control group but only a sixth of those in the treatment group. In addition, patients in the control group received home help between three and four times more frequently than those in the treatment group. Consequently, on average, patients in the control group received seven times as many visits from the home help services as those randomised to the nursing unit.

Since the dependency of patients in the two randomised groups did not differ significantly in the 6 months following discharge, it is surprising to find such a large discrepancy in frequency with which home help services were used. However, it is possible that the difference in the use of the home help services is related to the simultaneous increase in the life satisfaction of the patients randomised to Burford Nursing Unit and reflects a long-term benefit of the extra efforts and counselling it provides. In any case, such a large discrepancy in the demand for the Social Services need further examination.

The pilot study calculated that it appears that patients who were transferred to the nursing unit on average incurred costs which averaged £44.6 (3.4%) less than those who were allocated to the treatment group. If the probable cost of community care for the discharged treatment group patients were to be calculated, and combined with the reduced inpatient costs, it is reasonable to assume that the nursing unit is a very cost effective alternative to traditional Health Service facilities.

Although the Burford pilot study was on a small scale, with relatively few patients, it suggested the following general observations:

1. If the nursing in community hospitals was re-organised, they could be more effectively used as a means of reducing the length of patient stay in scarce acute hospital beds. In addition, referral of patients to a local hospital increases the value of that hospital to the community.
2. The average cost of treating patients randomised to the nursing unit was 3.4% less than the corresponding cost for patients randomised to the normal regime. Despite this, patients randomised to the nursing unit certainly fared no worse than patients randomised to other hospitals.
3. Patients admitted to (other) community hospitals had a longer stay in hospital, and cost more to treat, than patients randomised to the nursing unit.
4. The quality of nursing care provided by the nursing unit was well above average.
5. The hypothesis that nursing has a therapeutic contribution is supported by the fact that, 6 months after discharge, the life satisfaction of patients randomised to the nursing unit was significantly higher than that of patients randomised to a normal hospital ward.

The following recommendations were made from the pilot study:

1. This experiment should be repeated, on a larger scale, in a general hospital and with stricter randomisation to reduce any bias.
2. The nursing in community hospitals should be reorganised along the lines of those used in the nursing unit.
3. Policy and decision makers in the NHS should consider the implication of the underlying philosophy of the pilot study, in that nursing units appear to be cost effective.
4. Consideration should be given towards setting up and evaluating the success of nursing units in acute general hospitals.
5. Very much more emphasis should be placed on the effective use of good quality in-house research as a tool in the management of nursing and other resources within the NHS.

In conclusion, the results did support the research hypotheses and suggested that nursing beds could be a useful and effective addition to acute hospital services. However, as the sample size was small and the randomisation technique simple, no concrete conclusions could be drawn from the study. It was therefore evident that a larger study needed to be undertaken to attempt to validate these preliminary findings.

This study therefore became the pilot for a larger study. Although relatively small, it aroused great interest and support throughout the United Kingdom and enabled the research team to follow on to the major study with the confidence of having survived the 'mistakes and misconceptions' felt by many nurse researchers (Hockey, 1985).

3 | Literature Review

THE NEED FOR HEALTH CARE

Being 'healthy' is, says Mechanic (1975), a right of every individual, whilst achieving such a state in modern society is beocming less and less possible for its members. Western societies frequently view health in relation to disease (Friedson, 1975), with the 'healthy state' being seen as analogous to physiological homeostasis or the absence of 'disease'. The validity of such an assumption is strongly challenged by social scientists (e.g. Friedson, 1970, 1975; Field, 1972). Field asks if health is an objective state as defined by physicians or whether it is more a subjective state as perceived by individuals about themselves and influenced by societal values. He sees illness as a form of deviation from socially defined norms. Friedson describes this deviance as 'conduct which violates sufficiently valued norms'. Parsons (1951) defines health more positively, as 'the state of optimum capacity for the effective performance of valued tasks'.

Friedson (1975) sees the health care system as primarily a mechanism of social control to ensure isolation and treatment of ill members of society. Helt and Pelikan (1975) assert that current health care systems rarely provide a service which focuses on helping people come to terms with their own life events; promotes independence and enables consumers to make decisions about their own health. They suggest that medical intervention, though essential in acute illness, is over-emphasised in that it is seen as the only legitimate therapy, and as the indisputable leading discipline. Mechanic (1975) acknowledges that health care involves medical intervention, but asserts that good health and the recovery from illness often only peripherally depend on curative medicants provided by doctors.

13

Whilst prevailing ideologies see health care as legitimately revolving around medical intervention and the application of paramedical therapies, this is not inevitably so, says Tiffany (1977), who supports that health care can focus on helping people reach the 'state of optimum capacity' referred to in Parsons' (1951) definition of health.

Within British nursing, such radical sentiments about medicine and the paramedical therapies are not commonly expressed. Nurses and their leaders acknowledge the enormous contribution of these disciplines, and do not argue against the need for high level input of them into patient care. Current developments within nursing, however, consistently demonstrate a need for nursing to have a greater overall input into decision making in all health care settings and for nursing to be given a leading position for some client groups.

Whilst prevailing ideologies may well still place nursing in a position of subservience in relation to medicine and paramedical therapies, it is becoming apparent (or re-discovered) that nursing is more than maintaining people whilst therapists apply their therapy: it is therapeutic in itself. This is a major concept of the developing contemporary ideology of nursing.

CONTEMPORARY IDEOLOGY OF NURSING

Much development in the conceptual understanding of nursing has occurred in the last 20 years and there is a wealth of literature which reflects this. Currently, nursing is attempting to be clearer about the nature of its practice and the contribution it makes as a discipline in health care.

The most widely known attempt to define nursing is that of Henderson (1966):

> 'The unique function of the nurse is to assist the individual, sick or well, in the performance of those activities contributing to health or its recovery (or to a peaceful death) that he would perform unaided if he had the necessary strength, will or knowledge, and to do this in such a way as to help him gain independence as rapidly as possible.'

Many other attempts to clarify the nature of nursing have been made. Bower (1972) sees nursing as 'the application of knowledge to promote and maintain maximum health, comfort and care'. She also points out that nursing is unique amongst health professions in its property of being able to operate in a highly generalistic manner. Travelbee (1971) expands on this generalistic function and stresses the fact that nursing in hospitals occurs 24 hours a day.

A general acceptance of a humanistic approach is reflected in most recent literature, and nursing is most often seen as an essentially social activity. As such, the importance of developing relationships – both between nurses and patients, and between nurses and co-health workers – is usually seen as central to the nursing role. Chapman (1979) proposes that nursing is a 'social activity, an interactive process between individuals, the nurse and the patient', whilst Sundeen et al (1976) see the nurse as 'being involved with all the components of a person in a dynamic interaction.' La Monica (1979) says that the goal of nursing is 'to provide humanistic care adapted to individual needs.'

Contemporary nursing theory therefore asserts that nursing involves seeing the recipient as a holistic being and using this view to meet his or her individual needs through meaningful interaction. These assumptions usually form the basis of a range of conceptual models for nursing practice, designed to assist in curriculum development and in the delivery of nursing.

Roper (1976) purports that it is not possible to adequately describe what nursing is in a concise definition and argues that only a broad schematic explanation of an interpretation of nursing, presented in the form of a conceptual model, can give meaning to the reality of nursing. McFarlane states that such models are 'conceptual representations of reality' and are of use in developing nursing as a human service. Reilly (1975) considers conceptual models as essential in giving nurses 'a perspective way of looking at nursing.'

McFarlane asserts that the cure-oriented/medical-oriented model, pervasive routinisation and a rigid supervisory structure are inappropriate to nursing in any setting, and that the needs of individuals are not being met. Many nurses support this and give voice to the view that nurses should move from a medical model of practice to a model conceived for nursing through the analysis of what people need when they are ill, dependent, or unable to perceive how to achieve health (Riehl and Roy, 1980; Orem, 1980; Roper, 1979; Roper et al, 1980, 1981, 1983).

The recognition by many of the need to reform society's beliefs about the role of women led to a questioning of the subservience of nurses (mainly women) to doctors (mainly men) as well as the criticism of the power of medicine by social theorists (Friedson, 1975;). Nurses began to assert themselves and seek equality within the health care team. Batchelor (1980) lists a number of factors leading to this demand for equality: the changing status of women in society as a whole, the higher status of nurses as reflected by salaries; the enhanced quality of the entry to nurse training; the increased number of men in senior positions; and the rise in trade union movement by nurses.

Much of this drive for change in nursing emanates largely from nurses in leadership positions at the national level and those who became academics when nursing departments became established in the institutes of higher learning in the 1960s. The national nursing bodies exhort nurses to bring about a fairly radical practice change based on:

- Re-organising work patterns so that care is given by trained nurses and accountability to the patient is explicit (Marram et al, 1974; Pearson, 1983).
- Re-structuring of the nursing team so that the hierarchy is 'flattened' (Gonzalez, 1981).
- The development of a close relationship between nurse and patient, and involvement of the patient in planning care (Hall, 1964; Alfano, 1971).
- Basing practice on a model for nursing which incorporates the concept of holism (Smuts, 1926) and clarifies the contribution of nursing to health care (Roper et al, 1981; Pearson and Vaughan, 1984).
- The use of a problem-solving approach (Yura and Walsh, 1973; Marriner, 1979).

The amalgamation of these concepts is said to constitute a major reform in nursing (Pearson and Vaughan, 1984) and is frequently referred to as as the 'Nursing Process' by a vast array of nursing theorists and written about frequently in all of the major nursing journals. It can be said to represent the current ideology of nursing held by nursing's elite and leadership, and bringing it about in practice has become the concern of a number of initiatives by policy making bodies.

CONCEPTUAL MODELS FOR PRACTICE

McFarlane (1976) argues that all nurses should practice from a knowledge base which is sufficient to enable them to justify the actions they take and that professional nurses should base practice on a conceptual model. Conceptual models and theory develop-ment in nursing are somewhat confused in the literature. McFarlane (1976) comments on the 'utter semantic confusion' in theoretical nursing. She observes that nursing has a tendency to grasp at 'concrete, structural security too soon' and asserts that: 'like the world of the infant, the world of theory in nursing seems a "blooming, buzzing confusion".'

Johnson and Davis (1975) describe a conceptual model for nursing practice as a:

> 'systematically constructed, scientifically based, and logically related set of concepts which identify the essential components of nursing practice together with the values required in their use by the practitioner.'

This 'diagram', as it were, of what nursing is, provides for the nurse a diagnostic and treatment orientation for the specific practice of nursing (Riehl and Roy, 1980). The diagnosis and treatment refers to *nursing*, and not to the acts of medicine.

Riehl and Roy (1980) suggest that the current development of nursing models is a serious attempt to provide alternatives to the disease/medical/hospital-oriented models of the past and say that contemporary nursing, for the sake of patients, needs to develop models specific to nursing. They assert that, in using the 'Nursing Process' (Yura and Walsh, 1973) as a means to deliver nursing care, nurses have need of a conceptual model on which to base assessment, identification of patient problems, planning care, implementing care and evaluation of the outcomes.

Orem (1980) suggests that if nurses use the concepts and theories inherent in a model, they will practice more effectively and will be able to 'place in perspective, other descriptions of nursing including those in other areas of specialisation.'

Thus she, along with Roper (1976), believes that a satisfactory model will describe nursing in any context; it will have meaning to nurses in all specialities.

Orem (1980) goes on to observe that, through the emergence of models specifically for nursing, the nurse's role is:

'emerging from obscurity imposed by an over emphasis on the relationship between the physician and the nurse, and between employing institution and the nurse. Nurses are coming to recognise that an item of information about a patient may have one meaning for a physician, but quite a different meaning for the nurse.'

A number of models are described in the literature, and an attempt is made by Riehl and Roy (1980) to construct a unified model for nursing by amalgamating a variety of models. In their classification of models developed to date, they suggest that three types emerge: systems models, developmental models and interactionist models.

The basic premise of those nurses who favour a systems approach is the concept of an open system within an open system. Byrne and Thompson (1978) recommend that man be understood in the context of the subordinate systems of which he is composed, such as cell, organ and organ systems, and the superordinate systems in which he exists, namely the family, the community and the society.

Those nursing models which follow systems theory utilise the concept of man as an organism, existing in a steady state, being subjected to stress and then adapting or adjusting in order to re-establish its stability within the acceptable parametres. Orem (1980) and Roper et al (1980) both place extra emphasis on development and interaction, and, although systems based, expand the conceptualisation outside the narrower confines set by those theorists who attempt to pursue a purist system approach.

Other systems models include those of Bower (1977), Saxton and Hyland (1975), Neuman (1980) and Roy (1980).

Roper (1976, 1979) and Roper et al (1980, 1981, 1983) describe a model which incorporates many of the concepts inherent in the model described by Orem (1980) and the concept outlined by Henderson (1966).

Pearson and Vaughan (1986) report that agreement on a specific model within a nursing team gives direction to nursing work, and cohesion in care planning and giving. In a study of changing nursing norms, Pearson (1985) found that British nurses, when exposed to models, saw their relevance, but all generally favoured Roper et al's (1980) work because of its British origins. In the Pearson study, the selection of a model to direct practice led to a stronger nursing identity within the health team, and was seen as a precursor to the development of therapeutic nursing and the establishment of nursing beds (Pearson, 1987b).

NURSING BEDS

A number of nurses have argued that a need exists for the provision of hospital beds grouped into units which focus on the delivery of therapeutic nursing (e.g. Hall et al, 1975; Hall, 1966, 1969; Orem, 1966; Alfano, 1969, 1971; Poirer, 1975; Schaffrath, 1978; Pearson, 1983, 1985, 1987 a, b; Pearson et al, 1987). They all assert that patients in acute biological crisis require the services of an acute, high technology, medically led unit in the initial phases only and that as the crisis is lessened, the intensity of medical and paramedical intervention becomes lessened also. Both Alfano (1971) and Pearson (1983) suggest that as the crisis lessens, and the need for medical and paramedical intervention falls, the need for rehabilitative, nurturing nursing rises. They describe how post-crisis patients rapidly replace the need for medical care with a need for support, nurturing and teaching once the fear of death and/or pain is resolved, and that these latter needs are legitimately the concern of nursing. A study in 1975 involved the establishment of a nursing care unit and an evaluation of its effect on patient outcomes through the conduct of a controlled clinical trial (Hall et al, 1975). Those admitted to the nursing unit, when compared to those who pursued a 'normal' patient career in traditional facilities, were: re-admitted less; more independent; had a higher post discharge quality of life; and were more satisfied with their hospitalisation experience. A similar study in the United Kingdom (Pearson et al, 1987) produced strikingly similar results. As well as the apparent benefits for patients, the nursing units in both studies led to cost savings and to greater job satisfaction for nurses (Pearson, 1985), and there is evidence that giving nurses the opportunity to accept responsibility in units devoted to nursing as the primary mode of intervention leads to creative development of new methods of patient care and more effective use of time (Tutton, 1987; McMahon, 1986; Pearson, 1987b).

Both the Department of Health and Social Security (1980) and Batchelor (1980) concede that such beds need to be established for the elderly who require long-term, nursing home type care, and NHS nursing homes were established early in the 1980s in response to this identified need.

Nursing beds for post-crisis, acute patients have not, however, been generally seen as to be needed with the British NHS. The first such provision, established in a rural community hospital, was found to be effective, but not as accessible as it could have been were it placed within easy reach of an acute hospital (Pearson et al, 1987). The Royal College of Nursing suggests that the establishment of nursing beds in every health district in the United Kingdom would lead to higher quality of care (Clay, 1987).

NURSING AND NURSING BEDS

Nursing beds are essentially those established where 'nursing is the chief therapy and the nurse is the chief therapist' (Tiffany, 1977). They are based on the fundamental belief that nursing in itself can be therapeutic. Capra (1982) and Wilson-Barnett (1984) outline the therapeutic nature of nursing, and suggest that holistic care delivered by the nurse helps people to set realistic targets for change and supports them in reaching these targets. Kitson (1985) found, in her study of nursing elderly patients, that nursing has demonstrable therapeutic results in a range of areas (Davis, 1984; Wilson-Barnett, 1984; Boore, 1978; Hayward, 1975), and studies which evaluate the effect of teaching and interpersonal interaction by nurses on post-operative recovery all found measurable improvements in outcomes. Tutton (1987) reports improvement in feelings of comfort following the use of therapeutic touch by nurses and Egan (1975) reports intense therapeutic effects experienced by clients from skilled communication with nurses.

Travelbee (1971), Jourard (1971), Kitson (1985) and Krieger (1981) all suggest that nursing can be an effective therapeutic force and report on a wide range of studies to support this argument.

To operate therapeutically, nurses need authority to do so, and to possess high levels of skill in promoting physical and psychosocial comfort, communication and problem solving (Pearson and Vaughan, 1986; McMahon, 1986). Acute hospital wards limit authority. Because of their necessary focus on crisis intervention, constraints are imposed on the nurses who wish to practice holistically because the primary therapy is perceived to be medicine.

There is much evidence to suggest that therapeutic nursing is rarely practised in medically led, acute hopsital wards. Many empirical studies report that nursing focuses largely on meeting physical needs and that little attention is given to exploiting the therapeutic potential inherent in nursing someone (Norton et al,

1962; Stannard, 1973; Towell, 1975; Stockwell, 1972; Hawthorn 1974).

Pearson et al (1987) report that routinisation and rule following are inevitable because of the hierarchial structure of nursing, and Pearson (1985), in a study of nursing beds, found that organising nursing work through tasks or teams perpetuated the focus on physicality and that re-organising work so that certain nurses were responsible for a group of patients, promoted holistic care. Thus therapeutic care (referred to as primary nursing) had observable effects on improving the therapeutic content of nursing practice.

ADMISSION TO NURSING BEDS

The purpose of a nursing unit is to provide care for those who need professional nursing. Referral of patients will largely be done by doctors, as the need for intensive medical care rules out admission to the unit and medical assessment must preclude this need. Clinical nurse specialists, health visitors, District Nurses and others may initiate referral of patients should they identify specific nursing problems, but may need to channel the referral through the patient's own doctor for medical assessment. It is anticipated that the majority of referrals will be from doctors in the acute hospital setting or from GPs in the community. The reason for the referral must be the need for 'healing' nursing care (Pearson, 1983).

In the acute hospital setting, Hall (1963) and Alfano (1969) maintain that, as the need for intense medical care falls, the need for nursing rises. 'When a patient is in biological crisis, his chief concern is usually whether he will live or die. As the threat of death becomes less imminent, he becomes more actively involved in working through problems associated with regaining health and re-entering the world of active community living'. It is at this point that referral to the nursing unit may be desirable.

Hall (1964) outlines specific criteria for admission to a nursing unit. The patient must:

1. Be over 16 yeas of age (unless paediatric provision is made).
2. Require intensive nursing care in the intermediate setting (i.e. between hospital and home).

3.   Be recommended by his/her doctor (hospital consultant or GP).
4.   Be likely to be able to return to his or her own community.
5.   Be expected to stay in the unit for at least 1 week.

She suggests that the following must rule out admission to the unit. Patients should not be considered for admission if:

1.   Their return to the community is considered a physical, emotional, social improbability. If this is the case, nursing home care is indicated.
2.   They can return to the community directly from the hospital under an organised home care programme, such as District Nursing Services, etc.
3.   They can return to the community directly from the hospital under their own family auspices.
4.   They require intensive medical care and diagnostic work-ups. If this is the case, hospital admission is indicated.
5.   They constitute a hazard to the safety and health of others, and require special precautionary measures.
6.   If they are eligible for transfer to existing hospital facilities for longer term care, such as in the case of tuberculosis, rehabilitation, geriatrics, etc.

Hall (1964) emphasizes that the medical diagnosis of the patient is of less importance than his or her need for nursing.

Patients meeting the criteria can be referred by a doctor to the nurse in charge who would undertake a nursing assessment prior to discussing the patients with the unit admission team, which is comprised of a doctor attached to the unit, a social worker and other staff members when needed (Henderson, 1966), and a decision made. Discharge home would be on the basis of the achievement of the nursing objectives, the feelings of the patients and their families, and discussion with the community nursing services.

In some patients, it may be become apparent that they will no longer benefit from the NU's programme, but are still unable to manage at home. In such cases, after being brought to the highest level of function, the NU would arrange transfer to a nursing home, residential home or long-stay ward. Similarly, should the patient develop a condition which necessitates a need for high-level medical care, he or she would be transferred to a hospital.

PRIMARY NURSING

Manthey and Kramer (1970) first described the concept of primary nursing and later defined it as:

> 'a system for delivering nursing service that consists of four design elements: allocation and acceptance of individual responsiblity for decision making to one individual; individual assignment of daily care; direct communication channels; one person responsible for the quality of care administered to patients on a unit 24 hours a day, seven days a week.' (Manthey, 1980).

Tutton (1986), Pembrey (1984), Pearson (1983) and Sparrow (1986) all argue that primary nursing is the method of care delivery of choice, and suggest that its introduction should be encouraged.

Hegyvary and Haussman (1976) describe how primary nursing involves every patient being assigned a primary nurse who then cares for him/her throughout the hospital stay, when on duty, and delegates care to an associate nurse when off duty. Each primary nurse therefore carries a caseload of patients and is accountable for total care for those patients for the whole of the hospital stay. Marram et al (1974) reports significant improvements in patient outcomes in areas where primary nursing has been introduced and Daeffler (1975) found patients were more satisfied when nursed in a system of primary nursing.

THERAPEUTIC NURSING

Pearson (1985) suggests that therapeutic nursing, although possible and desirable in all settings where nursing takes place, can best be delivered in units where a nursing ideology can prevail; where nursing is perceived to be the primary therapeutic intervention; and where primary nursing is well established. The nursing unit established in this study was designed to fulfil these prerequisities and to accommodate post-crisis patients who frequently have a need for high-level nursing intervention. If nursing is in itself therapeutic in its effect, then it should, says Hall (1963), have an observable positive effect on recovery and quality of life when compared to 'caretaking' nursing which characterises, she asserts, nursing typically practised in acute, medically led units.

POST-CRISIS RECOVERY OF PATIENTS

Elderly patients recovering from a cardiovascular accident (CVA) comprise one typical group whose major need is for a high level of post-crisis nursing intervention and who are therefore amenable to transfer to the nursing unit.

Katz and Akpom (1976) claimed that measurement of primary socio-biological functions developed by him could be used to predict outcomes for stroke and hip fracture patients. Lind (1982), in a synthesis of seven studies of the effects of rehabilitation on stroke patients, suggested that functional gains by stroke patients are primarily attributable to spontaneous recovery. A major component of most of these rehabilitative regimes was physio-therapy, but rehabilitative nursing was also specified in at least three of the studies synthesized. An improvement of only one or two points in functional scoring recorded by Lehmann et al (1975) in one of the studies included in Lind's synthesis, was of disproportionate importance in that it could crucially affect discharge outcomes between remaining institutionalised or returning home. Achieving maximum independence in activities of daily living (ADL) is a major goal for therapeutic nursing intervention. Herman et al (1984) in a retrospective descriptive study of stroke patients in a community hospital in North America found that next to the level of clinical impairment, age and admission from home were the factors most likely to affect discharge home. In a British study, Graham and Livesey (1983) found that nearly 25% of admissions to a geriatric hospital during a 12 month period were readmissions. Readmission was most likely in the two weeks after discharge and was not related to age or livng arrangements, social problems, non-compliance of patient or inadequate rehabilitaton for 47% of readmissions.

In helping the patient to come to terms with chronic illness or disability, the nurse is seen as having a unique role both as co-ordinator of the interdisciplinary team and the primary deliverer of care (Bukowski et al, 1986).

Studies of patterns of urinary elimination (Rottkamp, 1985) and of self-medication (Taylor, 1984) both aim to increase indepen-dence levels by helping patients to achieve success in these areas. Egger and Stix (1984) promote a psychosomatic approach in the form of a semi-structured interview schedule to enable patients to come to terms with dependency and disability. Lawrence and

Christie (1979) studied patients who had suffered a stroke 3 years previously and found that 70% viewed their future with uncertainty or gloom. They found that people's response to disability was more important than physical disability *per se* and that 40% would have been helped by counselling. Ahlsiö et al (1984) similarly found that depression or anxiety were as important for quality of life as was physical disablement and that most patients recorded a deterioration in life satisfaction. A greater emphasis on psychosocial support was therefore needed in post-stroke rehabilitation. Studies in *Leisure after Stroke* (Sjögren, 1982) and *Predicting the Stroke Patient's Ability to Live Independently* (DeJong et al, 1982) also stressed the need to take account of social and environmental as well as physical and psychological factors in considering long-term outcomes for stroke patients.

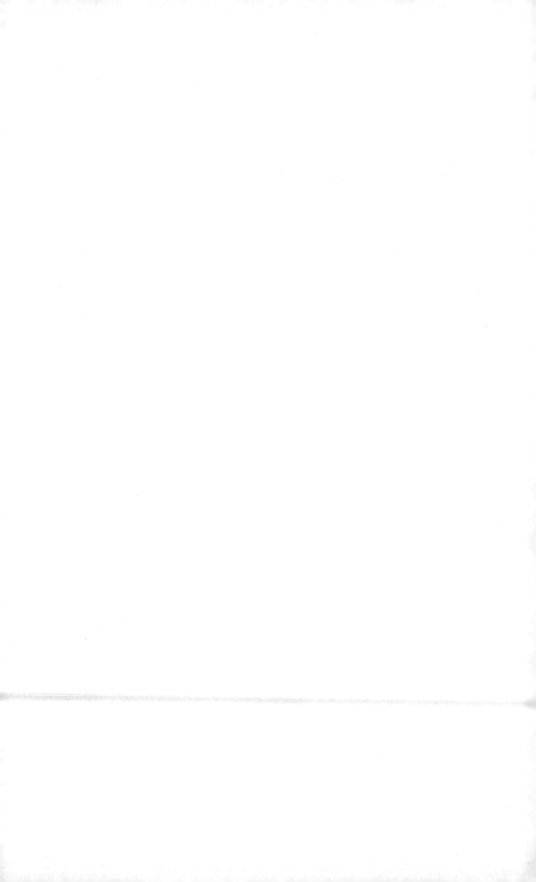

4 The nursing unit

'The Clinical Nursing Unit does not set out to propose that present day nursing care in hospitals is to be devalued, nor does it intend to duplicate the activities of other units!'
(Pearson, 1983)

'The Clinical Nursing Unit is needed when the primary need is teaching, counselling and nurturing which are inherent in professional nursing.'
(Hall, 1966)

The experimental nursing development unit on which this study reports was opened in September 1985. The idea grew from *The Clinical Nursing Unit* (Pearson, 1983) and the innovations made in the nursing unit involved in the pilot study. The nursing unit was to be the first in the United Kingdom to offer the service of 'nursing beds' within an acute general hospital while the philosophy of the unit was to be based on that of the Loeb Centre in New York.

The purpose of the nursing unit was to:

1. Admit and care for patients whose primary need was for intensive nursing.
2. Increase knowledge about the range of effectiveness of different nursing therapies.
3. Develop forms of nursing which facilitiate the involvement of patients as partners and increase the patients' knowledge and control of their own health.
4. Teach post-basic nurses advanced nursing practice.

LAYOUT

Supported by generous funding for the research by Monument Trust, the research team approached the Chief Nursing Officer of the Health Authority to seek a suitable site for a nursing unit. Three sites were offered and the nursing unit was established within an acute general hospital. The unit chosen had, up to 6 months previously, been an 18 bed elderly care ward which had been closed due to financial constraints. The physical layout appeared to have the most potential to create a therapeutic environment.

Funding was based on the cost of running 16 nursing beds, plus the cost of refurnishing, data collection and initial staff training. The ward offered a two-bed room, three single rooms and the main area divided into two-bed bays. The beds and bedside lockers remained, though all other furnishings were changed.

On opening, the nursing unit portrayed a homely atmosphere with fitted carpet in the vast sitting room, with a choice of seating in soft fabric or vinyl, a large dining table to enable family-type meal times, piano, television, a quiet library corner, and a bar for the patients and their visitors.

Beds were placed at varying angles with a pin board by each bed for patients to display cards, photographs, etc., creating a personal area for each patient. Many pictures, plants and collages brightened the walls. Verandas opening out from both sides of the ward were used in good weather. The nurses' station was situated centrally. In addition, the unit housed a seminar room with a library used for small meetings and study, and a staffroom for relaxation with coffee/tea making facilities. A large lecture room, seating approximately 30 people, was also attached for teaching and research activities. The unit offered an extensive clinical education programme to nurses and other health workers nationwide.

Primary nursing was chosen as the system for delivering nursing care and was practiced in its pure form as Manthey (1980) describes it (see Chapter 3).

The philosophy of the unit was based on the work of Lydia Hall. Hall (1966) presents her theory of nursing by drawing three circles which represent care, core and cure (Figure 4.1).

The Care circle represents the nurturing component of nursing and is exclusive to nursing. The professional nurse provides

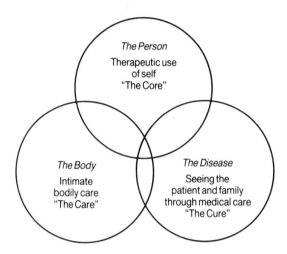

Figure 4.1 The person, the body, the disease.

bodily care for the patient, and helps complete such functions as eating, breathing and dressing.

The Core circle involves the therapeutic use of self and is shared with other members of the multidisciplinary team. The professional nurse, by developing a close relationship with her patients, is able to help patients express feelings regarding their illnesses and current health status.

The Cure circle is shared with other members of the multidisciplinary team, the nurse acting as an advocate of the patient and carrying out such activities as administering injections, etc.

These three aspects interact and the circles vary in size depending on the patient's progress. The nursing unit was designed to admit patients whose needs were predominantly for the care and core aspects of this concept (Figure 4.2).

In conjunction with the philosophy and primary nursing system the model of nursing used was the Roper et al (1980) model (Figure 4.3) based on the 12 activities of living, enabling the nursing process to be well established and documented.

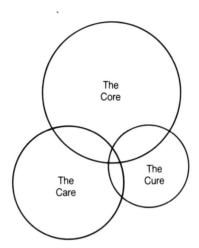

Figure 4.2 The care, the core, the cure.

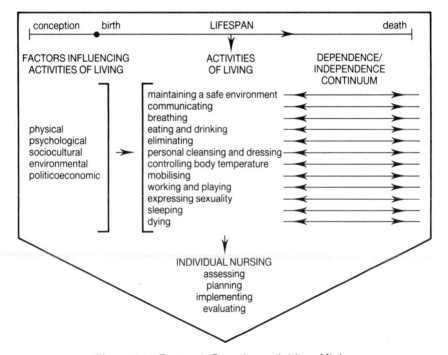

Figure 4.3 Factors influencing activities of living.

The model for nursing is based on a model of living and attempts to identify a concept of nursing to help nurses to develop a mode of thinking about nursing based on the process of living (see Chapter 3).

STAFFING

The nursing unit had two main objectives: first, to provide professional nursing care and, secondly, to test and generate nursing developments to bring more closely together nursing theory and practice. To achieve these objectives, selection of suitable staff was of paramount importance (Figure 4.4).

Establishment

Post	Whole time equivalent	Scale
Senior Nurse Practitioner	1.0	Sister I
Nurse Practitioner	2.0	Sister II
Associate Nurse	7.6	Staff Nurse
Ward Orderly	5.2	Anc III
Ward Co-ordinator	2.1	Clerical Officer
Activities Organiser	0.4	HCO
Medical Officer	0.26	Clinical Assistant

Figure 4.4 Staffing.

The positions were advertised nationally and locally, and the interview panel was made up of nurses with expertise in clinical nursing, research, education and management.

Only qualified nursing staff were employed. They had to be registered nurses with a belief in the unit philosophy, a sound clinical background and a good knowledge base.

The Senior Nurse Practitioner was the day-to-day manager of the unit, who acted as support nurse to the nurse practitioners and as an associate nurse to them, when necessary. On referral of a patient, she visited them in the acute setting to assess their nursing needs and suitability for transfer to the nursing unit. She was responsible for the planning and teaching of the clinical education programme, and acted as a research assistant.

The Nurse Practitioners, as primary nurses, were each

responsible for the holistic total nursing care of eight patients each, involving patients and their families in assessing needs and identifying problems; setting realistic objectives to be achieved; constructing a written plan of care; and implementing and evaluating this care. The nurse practitioners sought and acted upon the advice of nursing, medical, physiotherapy, occupational and social work advisors where appropriate. They were responsible for the discharge of their patients, sending a discharge summary to the GP. They had teaching commitments within the clinical education programme and were involved in research projects in clinical nursing.

Each practitioner had a team of Associate Nurses who carried out care and evaluated the written care plan when the practitioner was off duty. Full time associate nurses worked opposite shifts to their practitioner; evening and night associates completed the team. This ensured that each patient was cared for 24 hours a day by registered nurses, all of whom followed the same plan of care.

A linear rather than a hierarchical structure was used (see Figure 4.5).

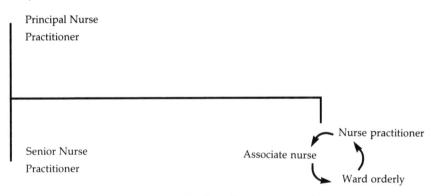

Figure 4.5   Staffing (linear structure).

In this structure the senior nurse practitioner acted as support nurse and consultant to the practitioners; the practitioners were accountable to their patients; the associate nurses were accountable to the patients for the care that they delivered and to the practitioner for implementing the care prescribed.

Ward Orderlies enabled the nursing to be delivered in this way. All direct nursing care was given by the nurse and the ward orderly performed mainly separate domestic duties (no separate domestic help was employed). The ward orderlies assisted nurses when 'two pairs of hands' were needed, but never gave direct care unsupervised. They completed such tasks as making unoccupied beds and preparing baths (tasks that have traditionally been done by nurses), allowing the nurse to remain at the bedside.

The Ward Co-ordinator acted as a ward clerk with extra responsibility, including office duties such as typing, photo-copying and filing. The use of 'walkie-talkies' facilitated quick communication between the co-ordinator and nurse practitioners which, again, freed the nurse to be with the patients.

The Activities Organiser provided activities and entertainment for patients on either an individual or group basis.

The Medical Officer had clinical responsibility for routine review and day-to-day medical cover as necessary, and was also responsible for medical review of patients referred to the nursing unit. Emergencies were covered by the on-call team within the hospital.

Physiotherapists, occupational therapists and social workers were involved and acted in consultative roles as experts in a multidisciplinary team meeting each week, and the medical advisor gave medical advice when his opinion was sought, once again in a consultative role.

ORIENTATION

Orientation of staff spanned 1 month, September–October 1985, and although involving the multidisciplinary team, it concentrated on nurses. In that time the principles and philosophy of the unit were discussed, developed and agreed. The professional theatre company, North West Spanner, worked with the team to promote good communication and counselling skills. This helped nurses to approach each patient as an individual and develop close relationships with them rather than imposing a directive way of care.

Two open days immediately prior to the official opening of the unit allowed visitors from all over the country to view the unit and question staff on the concept and running of the nursing unit.

The patient's day was completely individual, as was their nursing. Patients were encouraged to choose a routine they would normally follow at home, stating what time they wished to have breakfast, bathe and go to bed at night. Lunch and supper were shared with the two nurses on duty, allowing for a family-type occasion. Nurses and ward orderlies did not wear a uniform to encourage partnership in care rather than a directive approach. All patients, if capable, were taught self-medication. Education and teaching were emphasised, allowing patients to make informed choices in all aspects of their care. All nurses were skilled in massage techniques and aromatherapy, and incorporated this into their daily practice. Visiting hours were open and family participation encouraged.

Referral of patients to the unit was usually recommended by the ward sister or medical officer and approved by the appropriate consultant. Both the senior nurse practitioner and unit medical officer had power of veto on admission to the nursing unit (see Chapter 5).

The first patient was admitted to the nursing unit in October 1985.

5 Study design, procedure and methods

PURPOSE

The purpose of the study was to attempt to validate the findings of the pilot (Burford) study and in particular to test the following hypotheses:

- That care in the nursing unit will result in an independence level no lower than that achieved in other wards.
- That patients discharged from the nursing unit will be no less satisfied with the nursing care received than patients in other wards.
- That patients discharged from the nursing unit will have a level of satisfaction with life in general no lower than those discharged from other wards.
- That re-admission rates for patients discharged from the nursing unit will be no higher than those for patients discharged from other wards.
- That length of stay and/or cost per patient should be no longer/higher than for patients nursed on other wards.

METHODS AND PROCEDURE

The design of the study followed that of the pilot Burford study, but with a larger sample of patients and stricter randomisation.

The sample

The sample was to be drawn from patients of 60 years of age or over who had been admitted to the district general hospital with one of the following conditions:

- Fractured neck of femur.
- Cerebral vascular accident (CVA).
- Amputation of a lower limb.
- Abdominal hysterectomy.

As no patients in the last category were referred, the sample was limited to patients in the first three diagnostic groups.

Patients for inclusion in the study were referred by medical or nursing staff at the acute hospital as soon as their condition was considered stable enough for transfer. They were then assessed by a senior nurse, using a structured format incorporating the Clifton Assessment Procedure for the Elderly and also by the unit doctor for medical needs and clinical dependency (i.e. that no major medical condition existed which would require acute hospital care).

The purpose of the nursing assessment was to establish that a need for nursing existed and that discharge back into the community was a feasible possibility. To be included in the study, patients had to be sufficiently independent in the activities of living before admission to live in their own home or in Part III accommodation, and rational and oriented enough to understand what was happening to them and to answer questions about themselves.

Those patients who met these criteria were asked to give verbal consent to inclusion in the study (the consent of relatives might be obtained where appropriate) and they were then randomised, using a system of sealed envelopes numbered consecutively for 12 basic cohorts by age and sex in each diagnostic group. Inside each envelope was a card specifying whether the patient was in the control or treatment group. These cards derived from a computerised random numbers programme which attempted to ensure equal numbers of control and treatment patients for each diagnostic group.

Because not as many patients were referred as had been expected, in some groups the full complement of envelopes was not used, so that a matching number of control and treatment patients was not achieved in every category. In other groups the envelopes were exhausted before the end of the study and further envelopes were prepared, up to a total of 310.

The randomisation procedure was carried out in accordance with a strict protocol, envelopes being opened in numerical order by age, sex and diagnosis. Once randomised, treatment group patients were transferred to the nursing unit as soon as was practicable. Control patients followed the normal course of hospitalisation, either remaining in the acute hospital until discharge or being transferred to a community hospital.

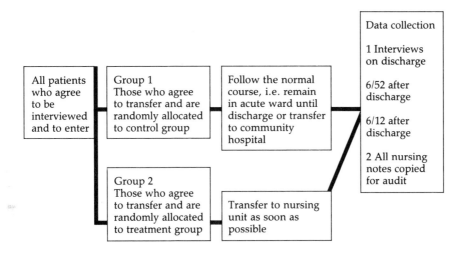

Figure 5.1   The study design.

Data collection – research tools

Nursing audit scores
Nursing notes were to be obtained for all sample patients and audited after discharge by a senior nurse from the Department of Geriatrics using the same criteria as for the district quality control (Pearson, 1987a).

Notes for all patients in the treatment group were automatically sent for audit. For the control group, however, it sometimes proved difficult to retrieve copies of the nursing notes, especially where the patient was transferred to a community hospital.

Because the nursing unit had its own record forms, it was possible to discern between control and treatment groups when auditing. The nurse auditor was confident, however, that there was no bias in the results.

Interview schedules

Data were obtained from patients by personal interview using the same schedule as in the pilot study, administered by a research assistant.

Patients were interviewed on discharge from hospital (within 24 hours whenever possible), and again 6 weeks and 6 months after discharge. The last two interviews took place wherever the patient was then living (i.e. in their own home, in residential accommodation or a nursing home).

The schedule for the first interview consisted of:

- An initial patient history (completed from patient records) and other biographical data.
- The nursing dependency index modified as in the pilot study (Garroway et al, 1980).
- A life satisfaction profile (Neugarten et al, 1961) which included a measure of social activity (Hall et al, 1975).
- A patient service checklist (Pearson et al, 1987).

The overall schedule was found by the research assistant to be, on the whole, appropriate. However, if the patients were not rational, or were confused, it was not possible to get answers to all the questions. Relatives and carers were therefore involved in such cases.

The extent to which professional support services were used after discharge was assessed by patients who noted each time that they were visited by the social services, and which social service was involved, on cards provided especially for this purpose.

There was some modification to the interview schedules because of these reasons. In the 'Satisfaction with care and basic biographic schedule', a question relating to the patient's religion was found to be irrelevant and it was thence removed.

A question in the initial patient history of the Nursing Dependency Scale that related to the source of admission was modified. An additional category was inserted for the patients admitted from institutional care, since some patients would be admitted from Part III or nursing homes. The 'activities of living' was found to be quite problematic, which was probably due to the fact that it was designed for patients who had suffered a cerebral vascular accident. Modifications were made to this to accommodate the nature of the patients in this study.

The main problem was in the definition sheet which accompanied the nursing dependency index and modifications were made to the function sheet as follows:

Function – feeding: this function seemed to resemble too closely the previous function of the provision of meals. The definitions were thus altered to give five graded performances. The first was altered to read 'to eat a full meal without aids or person'; the second to 'able to eat meals using prescribed aids such as plate walls, non-slip mats, special cutlery'; the third, 'requires the assistance of one person to cut food, can then use cutlery'; the fourth, 'dependent on two people to lift or position for feeding'; and the fifth, 'totally dependent for feeding, unable to feed self at all'.

Function – communication, speech and comprehension: this function was deemed irrelevant to the study, and omitted from the definition sheet.

Function – sleep: the third definition was altered from 'wakes once or twice during the night for toilet purposes, able to attend to own requirements' to 'unable to attend to own requirements'. The fourth definition of 'requires attention during the night for toilet purposes, able to sleep well afterwards' was modified to 'requires attention during the night for toilet purposes, needs the help of two people'.

These minor modifications were made prior to the commencement of this study.

The second interview schedule omitted the first and fourth points above but included a series of open-ended questions designed to elicit spontaneous comment on patients' experiences in hospital; the third interview schedule included only one open-ended question, but was otherwise identical to the second.

All the schedules are reproduced in the Appendix.

Information from records
Data on length of stay and destination on discharge were derived from records. Data on re-admissions was not collected systematically because of problems of retrieval and were therefore incomplete.

Data on costs forms the subject of Chapter 8.

A research assistant was responsible for administering the questionnaire and for recording all patient information on the schedules.

Data analysis

The data were coded for computation and the raw data transferred to the computer.

Quantifiable data were analysed by computer, using the Statistical Package for the Social Sciences (SPSS).

Qualitative data, including spontaneous comments where relevant, were transcribed and categorised on the basis of common themes.

LIMITATIONS OF THE STUDY

All social research is liable to certain limitations by virtue of the fact that its subject is human activity, which is almost by definition individualistic and unpredictable, resisting classification and deductive proof. The present study was no exception and, in addition, suffered from other limitations of which the research team was aware (some of which have already been mentioned in outlining the study procedure).

The study was designed to test the results of the pilot study on a larger sample. One of the problems which soon became apparent was the slow rate of patient referral for the sample. Reasons for this may have included misunderstanding about the nature of the study on the part of nursing staff, and certainly involved some opposition to the philosophy of nursing underpinning the study on the part of some senior clinicians and other medical staff. Every effort was made at a personal and a conceptual level, by senior nurses from the nursing unit who waged a constant propaganda battle with some of their colleagues. Nevertheless the size of the final sample was smaller than had been hoped. A larger sample would, of course, have yielded more information and more reliable evidence.

There was also a loss of data when sample patients had to be withdrawn from the study. This happened if treatment group patients had to be re-admitted to the acute hospital or if control patients were discharged before the initial interview and carers felt they could not, at that stage, cope with a visit from a researcher. On principle, no patient who wished to withdraw was over-persuaded to continue and this led to a further small loss of data. (Having said this, a response rate of 95.7% was achieved at first interview which was not unsatisfactory.)

Further unnecessary withdrawals took place before the second interview, at 6 weeks after discharge, owing to a policy change regarding re-admissions. Initially it was decided that patients re-admitted to hospital for any reason after discharge interview would not be interviewed again. When it was realised that this might exclude a considerable number of study patients, it was decided that interviews should continue with re-admitted patients, even though their nursing dependency and life satisfaction scores might not be comparable with those patients who had continued to make progress after discharge. Several 6 week and 6 month interviews were carried out subsequently in hospital once this change in policy had been agreed. In fact the very last patient to be interviewed for the study, a male with a fractured neck of femur, was bedfast in an orthopaedic hospital at the time of the third interview 6 months after his initial discharge, having suffered complications which eventually necessitated a hip replacement.

Problems were also experienced with some of the data collection tools, even though these had already been tested in the pilot study. In particular, the patient service checklist (which originated in the United States) proved difficult to administer, especially coming at the end of an already long interview. Respondents also sometimes exhibited a natural desire to please for fear of reprisals?) which may have influenced the answers given. This same tendency was sometimes suspected with the life satisfaction index.

The research was based on the assumption that the experience of being nursed in the unit was the dependent variable. This could not, of course, be proved, as many extraneous factors were also at work. In particular it is at least possible that patients' inborn characteristics and the habits and experience of 60 years of life may have been at least as effective in promoting recovery or its opposite as any method of nursing. Even if it were proved that the type of nursing care given to the patient was the dependent variable influencing recovery, there is still the possibility of the influence of the Hawthorn effect which states that any modification of the *status quo* in an institutional setting is likely to bring about improvement.

Finally, there is the question of interviewer bias. All but a tiny fraction of interviews were conducted by the same research assistant who was based at the nursing unit. Consistency in data collection and recording was thus reasonably assured, but not interviewer impartiality. As the initial interview nearly always took place before discharge, the location made it unavoidable that the interviewer knew to which group the patient being interviewed belonged. Indeed it was her responsibility to keep track of control group patients who were frequently transferred between wards at the acute hospital or to community hospitals.

Awareness of the possibility of bias was the first answer to this problem. The research assistant who carried out the interviewing had previous experience as an interviewer. Her training and background were in social science and, not being a nurse herself, she carried few preconceptions about different philosophies of nursing, which minimised the risk of attachment to any one school of thought. Although based at the nursing unit, she did not spend long periods of time there and, as far as was consistent with good manners, adopted a policy of not becoming involved socially with patients before their discharge.

At the later interview, interest in the welfare and progress of each patient individually tended to outweigh other considerations.

6 Results – quantifiable data

THE STUDY SAMPLE

A total of 164 patients were randomly assigned to either the treatment group (87) or a control group (77). Three patients assigned to the treatment group were withdrawn; one did not wish to participate; and two were re-admitted to an acute care hospital prior to the first interview. Similarly, four of those assigned to the control group were withdrawn from the study; three did not wish to participate; and one was transferred out of the area covered by the health authority. This resulted in 84 patients in the treatment group and 73 in the control group (Table 6.1).

Table 6.1 The study sample

	Treatment	Control	Total
Initial Random Assignment	87	77	164
Withdrawals from sample:			
refused	(1)	(3)	(4)
transferred	—	(1)	(1)
re-admitted to ACU	(2)	—	(2)
Total remaining	84	73	157

Attrition

Patient deaths and re-admissions to hospital resulted in the loss of some data: a breakdown of the number of completed interviews at each stage of data collection is shown in Table 6.2. Some records are incomplete because patients were confused or disoriented during the interviews and unable or unwilling to respond to the interview questions.

Table 6.2 Sample attrition

	Treatment	Control	Total
Total for study	84	73	157
Died before first interview	(6)	(15)	(21)
Total remaining	78	58	136
Completed first interview	74	50	124
Withdrawals prior to second interview			
refused	(1)	(1)	(2)
moved out of area	(1)	—	(1)
re-admitted to ACU	(3)	—	(3)
other	(2)	—	(2)
died before second interview	(4)	(3)	(7)
Completed second interview	63	46	109
Completed third interview	58	41	99

DEMOGRAPHIC CHARACTERISTICS

Data on selected demographic variables are shown in Table 6.3. There were more women (61%) than men (39%) in the group. About a third of the participants were married (33%) and half were widowed (51%). The majority were last employed over 5 years ago (77%) and had a secondary school education (82%). Approximately one half of the group lived in a house prior to entering hospital. Similarly, about one half of the study participants lived alone prior to hospitalisation. There was a significant relationship ($p<0.001$) between living situation (alone or with others) and marital status, with over 74% of the widowed patients living alone. Living situation was not related to sex or type of residence.

Table 6.3 Demographic characteristics of study participants

	Total sample n (%)
Sex	
male	61 (38.9)
female	96 (61.1)
Marital status	
never married	18 (14.0)
married	42 (32.6)
widowed	66 (51.2)
other	3 (2.3)
missing	28
Living situation	
with others	73 (51.0)
living alone	70 (49.0)
missing	14
Residence	
house	62 (49.2)
bungalow	24 (19.0)
flat	15 (11.9)
warden controlled	13 (10.3)
part III accommodation (i.e. hostels)	6 (4.8)
other	6 (4.8)
missing	31
Last employed	
less than 5 years ago	14 (12.8)
5+ years ago	84 (77.1)
never worked	11 (10.1)
missing	48
Education	
secondary school	78 (82.1)
grammar school	11 (11.6)
college/university	6 (6.3)
missing	62

Breakdowns of the demographic data by group are shown in Table 6.4. The treatment and control groups were similar in terms of demographic characteristics, indicting that the randomisation procedure was effective.

Table 6.4 Breakdown of selected demographic variables by group

	Treatment group n (%)	Control group n (%)
Sex		
male	35 (41.7)	26 (35.6)
female	49 (58.3)	47 (64.4)
Marital status		
never married	7 (9.1)	11 (21.2)
married	27 (35.1)	15 (28.8)
widowed	42 (54.5)	24 (46.2)
other	1 (1.3)	2 (3.8)
missing	7	21
Living situation		
with others	39 (48.8)	34 (54.0)
living alone	41 (51.3)	29 (46.0)
missing	4	10
Residence		
house	36 (48.0)	26 (51.0)
bungalow	19 (25.3)	5 (9.8)
flat	9 (12.0)	6 (11.8)
warden controlled	8 (10.7)	5 (9.8)
part III accommodation (i.e. hostels)	2 (2.7)	4 (7.8)
other	1 (1.3)	5 (9.8)
missing	9	22
Last employed		
less than 5 years ago	6 (9.0)	8 (19.0)
5+ years ago	55 (82.1)	29 (69.0)
never worked	6 (9.0)	5 (11.9)
missing	17	31
Education		
secondary school	50 (83.3)	28 (80.0)
grammar school	7 (11.7)	4 (11.4)
college/university	3 (5.0)	3 (8.6)
missing	24	38

The ages are normally distributed around a mean of 80.7 years with a standard deviation of 6.8 years. The mean age of males (78.3 years) was significantly lower ($p<0.001$) than the mean age of females (80 years). There was no significant difference in the mean age of the treatment and control groups which were 80.4 and 80.9 years respectively.

MEDICAL DIAGNOSIS

The medical diagnosis of the participants admitted to hospital were categorised as:

- 88 patients or 56% were admitted following a CVA;
- 62 patients or 39% suffered a fractured neck of femur; and
- 7 patients or 15% were admitted for amputation of a lower limb.

A breakdown of medical condition by group is provided in Table 6.5; the distribution of patients in the treatment and control groups with different medical diagnoses did not differ statistically.

Table 6.5 Breakdown of medical diagnoses by group

Diagnosis	Treatment group n (%)	Control group n (%)
Fracture	35 (41.7)	27 (37.0)
CVA	45 (53.6)	43 (58.9)
Other	4 (4.8)	3 (4.1)
Total	84 (100.1)	73 (100.0)

The mean CAPE scores are given by group for each diagnosis in Table 6.6. There were no significant differences in CAPE scores for the treatment and control groups. Similarly there were no significant differences between the two groups when t-tests were undertaken for each diagnosis.

Table 6.6 Mean CAPE scores by medical diagnosis and group

Diagnosis	Treatment group (n = 84) mean (S.D.)	Control group (n = 73) mean (S.D.)
Fracture	12.2 (4.4)	12.4 (4.2)
CVA	11.6 (4.3)	13.4 (4.6)
Other	8.3 (1.0)	16.7 (7.2)
Total	11.7 (4.4)	13.2 (4.6)

There were significant relationships between medical diagnosis and age. Patients hospitalised following a CVA had a mean age of 79 years compared with a mean age of 83 years for those with a fractured neck of femur.

While there were equal numbers of men and women admitted following a CVA, there were significant differences in the sex distribution for the other two diagnoses. For a fractured neck of femur there were 51 women compared with only 11 men admitted, while for amputations there were six men compared with only one women.

TIME SPENT IN ACUTE CARE AND UNDER NHS CARE

The length of hospital stay for the treatment and control patients is shown in Table 6.7. In keeping with the study design, patients selected for transfer to the nursing unit spent significantly less time in the acute care hospital, with a mean acute care stay of 10.8 days compared to 33.7 days for the control patients. The distribution of days spent in acute care is shown for the control patients in Figure 6.1 and for treatment patients in Figure 6.2. As can be seen, in both groups the average stay figures are affected by patients with extremely long hospitalisations. However, even allowing for the effect of the extreme cases, the treatment patients spent significantly less time in the acute care hospital than did the control patients ($p<0.001$).

Table 6.7 Length of hospital stay by hospital and group

Hospital	Treatment group (n = 80) mean (S.D.)	Control group (n = 63) mean (S.D.)
ACU	10.8 (9.2)	33.7 (29.0)
Beeson unit	36.6 (25.0)	NA
Community hospital (n = 16)	NA	35.9 (30.6)
Total number of days	47.2 (27.5)	42.9 (32.8)

The average number of days under NHS care differed slightly for the two groups, with mean total stays of 47.2 and 42.9 days for the treatment and control patients respectively; however, this

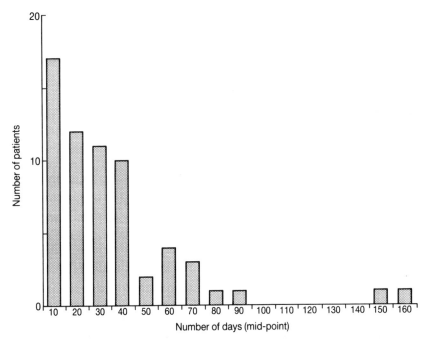

Figure 6.1 Days in acute care (control)

difference was not statistically significant. In both groups, small numbers of patients had extremely long hospitalisations (see Figures 6.3 and 6.4).

A breakdown of stay in acute care units by group and diagnosis is shown in Table 6.8. Analysis of variance indicated that the main effects of both group ($p<0.001$) and diagnosis were significant ($p<0.001$). In addition, there was a group/diagnosis interaction ($p<0.01$). The main effect of group supports the analysis indicating

Table 6.8 Days in acute care beds by group and diagnosis

| Diagnosis | Treatment group | | | Control group | | | Total |
	n	mean	(S.D.)	n	mean	(S.D.)	mean (S.D.)
Fracture	35	7.6	(6.0)	25	18.7	(10.3)	12.3 (9.7)
CVA	41	11.9	(8.5)	35	44.1	(34.3)	26.7 (28.8)
Other	4	26.3	(20.5)	3	37.0	(14.0)	30.9 (17.6)
Total	80	10.8	(9.2)	63	33.7	(29.0)	

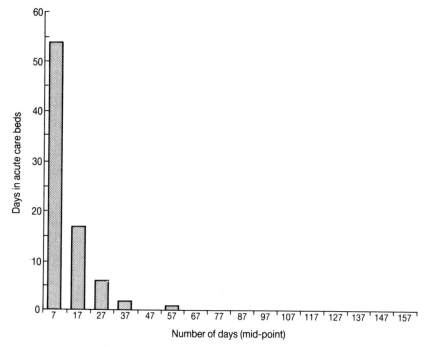

Figure 6.2   Days in acute care (treatment)

that treatment patients spent less time in acute care beds than did control patients (Figure 6.5). The main effect of diagnosis suggests that patients with a fractured neck of femur spend less time in acute care than patients with a CVA. The interaction effect appears due to the extremely long acute care hospital stays experienced by some CVA patients in the control group.

A similar breakdown of total days under NHS care is shown in Table 6.9. Analysis of variance indicates that there was no significant effect of group demonstrating that treatment and control patients did not differ in the total amount of time spent in hospital. There was, however, a significant effect of diagnosis ($p < 0.01$), suggesting patients with a CVA spend longer in NHS care than do patients with a fractured neck of femur (Figure 6.6). There was also a significant group/diagnosis interaction ($p < 0.01$), which in this instance appears due to the relatively short stay of control group patients with a fractured neck of femur (mean = 27.9 days) compared with the stay durations of control group patients with a CVA (mean = 53.7 days) and treatment patients

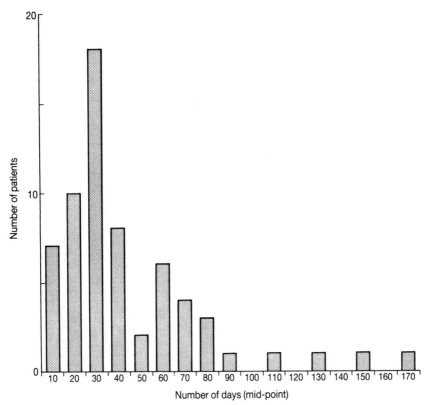

Figure 6.3 Total days, NHS (control)

Table 6.9 Total days in NHS care by group and diagnosis

Diagnosis	Treatment			Control			Total	
	n	mean	(S.D.)	n	mean	(S.D.)	mean	(S.D.)
Fracture	35	43.5	(28.1)	25	27.9	(34.9)	37.0	(27.9)
CVA	41	48.9	(27.2)	35	53.7	(34.9)	51.1	(30.9)
Other	4	62.3	(24.5)	3	41.7	(22.0)	53.4	(24.2)
Total	80	47.2	(27.5)	63	42.9	(32.8)		

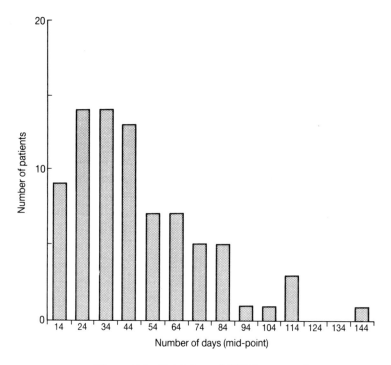

Figure 6.4 Total days, NHS (treatment)

with a fractured neck of femur and patients with a CVA (means of 43.5 and 48.9 days respectively).

QUALITY OF NURSING CARE

The quality of nursing care was assessed using the nursing audit review schedule. Total scores and scores on each of the seven subscales for treatment and control patients are shown in Table 6.10. Quality of care in the nursing unit was rated significantly higher on each of the subscales. Using a Mann–Whitney test all subscales were significantly higher at the 0.1% level. Similarly, the total quality of care score was significantly higher for the nursing unit patients than for the control patients ($p < 0.001$).

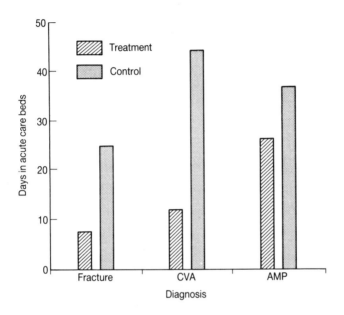

Figure 6.5 Means days, acute care, by group & diagnosis

DEATHS IN HOSPITAL AND RESIDENCE AFTER DISCHARGE

Information on patient deaths in hospital and on where patients went after discharge is shown in Table 6.11. In all, 54% of the patients were discharged to their homes. Outcomes of the hospital stay for the two groups differed statistically ($p<0.05$), with proportionately more treatment patients than control patients discharged home, and proportionately less treatment patients than control patients dying in hospital. Of 21 deaths in hospital, 18 were patients with a cerebral vascular accident (13 control, five treatment). The number of patients who died in hospital differed significantly, as shown in Table 6.11a.

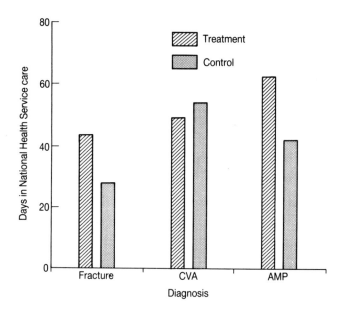

Figure 6.6 Means days, NHS, by group & diagnosis

There were some difficulties tracing the records of those patients who had died in hospital. The outcome of these difficulties is that the data that has been considered in the preceding tables includes seven patients who died in hospital (Table 6.11b). Two of these patients were from the treatment group and five were from the control group.

NURSING DEPENDENCY

Scores on the nursing dependency inventory are shown for each group in Table 6.12. When discharged from hospital (the time of the first interview), the treatment patients were more able to perform activities of daily living than were the control patients ($p<0.01$). By the time of the second interview, conducted 6 weeks after discharge, the dependency scores of the control group had

Table 6.10 Nursing audit scores by group

Part II: Nursing Audit Chart review schedule Section heading (max score)	Treatment (n = 64) mean (S.D.)		Control (n = 22) mean (S.D.)	
1. Application and execution of physician's orders (42)	37.1	(5.6)	30.2	(6.8)
2. Observation of symptoms and reactions (40)	37.9	(2.7)	28.7	(8.2)
3. Supervision of the patient (28)	27.4	(1.4)	17.1	(7.2)
4. Supervision of those participating in care (20)	19.9	(0.8)	11.1	(5.4)
5. Reporting and recording (20)	18.9	(1.7)	14.3	(4.1)
6. Application and execution of nursing procedures (32)	29.3	(3.1)	23.7	(3.2)
7. Promotion of physical and emotional health (18)	17.3	(1.3)	9.1	(5.6)
Final score	187.5	(8.2)	131.2	(31.8)

Table 6.11a Residence after discharge and deaths in hospital, by group

	Treatment group n (%)	Control group n (%)
Home	55 (65.5)	30 (41.1)
Private home	13 (15.5)	12 (16.4)
Other	9 (10.7)	6 (8.2)
Died in hospital	6 (7.1)	15 (20.6)
Remaining in acute care	—	10 (13.7)
Missing	1 (1.2)	—

Table 6.11b Analysis of patient deaths in hospital, by group

Significance	Treatment group	Control group	chi squared
Died in hospital	6	15	$X^2 = 6.06$
Discharged/remained in hospital	78	58	$p < 0.05$

dropped to the same level as those of the treatment patients. Mean ratings of dependency remained stable through the 6 month interview and the two groups did not differ (Figure 6.7).

Table 6.12 Nursing dependency scores by group

| | Treatment group | | | Control group | | |
	n	mean	(S.D.)	n	mean	(S.D.)
First interview	74	39.7	(8.1)	50	43.8	(8.6)
Second interview	63	38.4	(12.4)	46	39.3	(11.6)
Third interview	58	38.8	(13.1)	41	37.8	(11.6)

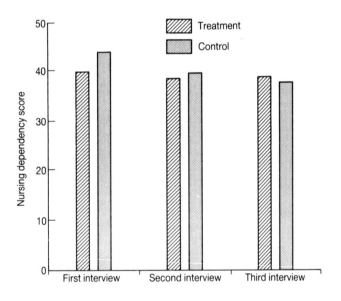

Figure 6.7 Nursing dependency scores by group

Mean scores on the 'requiring human assistance' component of the nursing dependency inventory are shown for each group in Table 6.13. The results show a pattern like that of the overall scores: higher needs for assistance in the control group at discharge with a drop to treatment group levels at 6 weeks. Again the treatment patient scores remain unchanged from discharge to 6 months (Figure 6.8).

Table 6.13 Requiring human assistance scores by group

	Treatment group			Control group		
	n	mean	(S.D.)	n	mean	(S.D.)
First interview	74	24.6	(12.5)	50	31.2	(13.9)
Second interview	63	23.2	(17.8)	46	24.5	(17.4)
Third interview	57	24.2	(17.8)	40	23.5	(16.2)

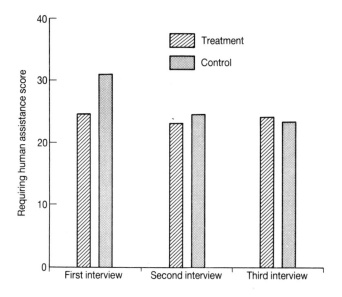

Figure 6.8 Requiring human assistance by group

LIFE SATISFACTION

Mean scores on the life satisfaction scale are shown for each group in Table 6.14. There were no differences between the treatment and control patients on this measure of life satisfaction at any of the three interviews. Overall there was a significant decline in life satisfaction scores between the first and the second interviews ($p < 0.05$). Life satisfaction scores were not related to medical diagnosis (Figure 6.9).

Table 6.14 Life satisfaction scores by group

	Treatment group			Control group		
	n	mean	(S.D.)	n	mean	(S.D.)
First interview	64	40.0	(6.3)	40	38.4	(6.1)
Second interview	51	37.0	(5.9)	37	37.4	(6.2)
Third interview	38	38.6	(6.0)	29	38.1	(5.9)

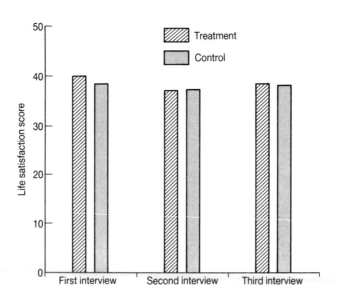

Figure 6.9 Life satisfaction scores by group

PATIENT SATISFACTION WITH CARE – PATIENT SERVICES CHECK LIST

Scores on the patient service check list are shown in Table 6.15. The possible scores range from 0 to 92, and questions marked as not applicable were scored using the mean score of the answered items.

Table 6.15 Patient service check list: analysis of total score by group

Group	Mean score	Standard deviation	t-test
Control ($n=32$)	74.61	13.60	$t = -2.50$
Treatment ($n=58$)	81.45	10.00	$p < 0.02$

As with the nursing audit scores, the variability in the control group scores was greater than that of the treatment group scores ($p<0.05$). A *t*-test performed using separate variance estimate indicates that the mean treatment group score was significantly greater than the mean control group score.

7 Results – qualitative data

THE EXPERIENCE OF INTERVIEWING

The research hypotheses (see Chapter 5) involved some measures of patient satisfaction (with life in general and with the nursing care received) which were subjective and not amenable to statistical analysis. The method of data collection, by personal interview, was also to some extent an exercise in subjectivity, despite the use of closed question schedules. Some account of the interviewer's experience may therefore complement the presentation of objective data and precede a discussion of the qualitative data.

Place of discharge was recorded at the initial interview. About a week before the second interview was due, contact would be made, either by phone or by sending a standard letter suggesting a date and time for the inteviewer to visit, which had the advantage of reminding the person concerned that they had agreed to take part in the research (and very few remembered anything about it!) and might be followed up by a phone call. In other cases, especially with those living nearby, a visit might be made unannounced, but always a full explanation was given and identity disclosed before entry. In the case of patients discharged to residential care, staff were contacted by telephone beforehand.

Very few patients refused co-operation and many welcomed a visit from 'the hospital', frequently expressing gratitude that anyone should show an interest in them. The fact that the research 'had nothing in it for them', the researcher had not come to offer any assistance and respondents were sometimes upset by some of the questions, did not seem to diminish this feeling and, where it existed, this certainly made the interviewer's job easier.

61

Some were less co-operative, refusing to answer the same 'damned silly questions' over again.

Patients were seen in their own or relatives' homes, in Part III accommodation and private nursing homes. Occasionally interviews took place in hospital, which had some advantages. It solved problems of access and staff could usually provide reliable information, such as on nursing dependency level. In at least one case it certainly enabled the respondent to talk more freely than when his rather over-protective wife was present at home. On the other hand, severely dysphasic patients had difficulty in answering the more open-ended questions and the presence of a spouse would then have been useful.

When patients were in residential care, staff were invariably helpful and data on nursing dependency was obtained or at least checked with staff. Usually the interview was in private (often in the dining room at a table already laid for the next meal) but sometimes, especially in Part III accommodation, it had to be conducted in the lounge, and usually in a loud voice because of deafness and competition from the television. These were some of the more dispiriting encounters. Where patients were confused, the views of staff were recorded and the later interviews might then be done by telephone but every patient was seen at least once, though on one occasion the 'interview' consisted of looking at pictures in a magazine in an attempt to gain some slight response.

Deafness caused some problems, but these could be overcome in a one-to-one situation except with the more complex life satisfaction index and the open-ended questions. Dysphasic patients who had suffered a stroke were perhaps the most difficult to communicate with and one sensed the tide of frustration which threatened to overwhelm a highly intelligent man unable to make himself understood or liable to say 'yes' when he meant 'no'.

A handful of patients attempted to manipulate the interviewer, to obtain benefits although it was made clear she had no power to give them. When a genuine request for specific help was made, the non-participant role of the interviewer was explained, but wherever possible some co-operation was offered. For example, several treatment group patients were referred back to staff at the unit and control patients were put in touch with social workers or speech therapists. Practical help included form filling and transporting unwanted aids-to-daily-living back to hospital. It was even proved that a wheelchair could be fitted in the back of a mini!

Interviewer bias has already been discussed, but one problem arose when treatment group patients asked about the nursing unit – and several were genuinely interested in its progress. One man even contacted the local radio station because he felt it so important that more people should know about the unit, which resulted in an article about him in the local press! Individual nurses and also ward orderlies were asked after by name, and although these conversations nearly always took place after the end of the formal interview, no comparable discussion about their hospital experience was possible with control patients. Nevertheless the impression was given, especially in the earlier stages of the study, that the unit induced in some patients warm and supportive feelings which were expressed in terms such as 'homely', 'friendly' or 'family atmosphere'. A similar reaction was recorded from one or two of the patients who had been nursed at one particular community hospital. They, too, remembered nurses (and also other patients) by name and the husband of one described it as 'the best thing that happened [in the community hospital] for a long time'.

In the course of the three interviews a degree of rapport was established with most of the respondents, even when the initial response had been hostile or indifferent. One dysphasic woman chose to vent her frustration at her continuing speech problems and depression on the hospital and (as she saw it) its representative but mellowed on finding that her criticisms were taken seriously and when a mutual interest was discovered. She became so friendly that it was difficult to conclude the interview. It would be wrong to give the impression that all the respondents were unfailingly friendly and open in their answers; however, many undoubtedly were, and the fact that some of the impressions formed in the course of the 22 month period of interviewing had been confirmed by the analysis of qualitative data, gives some confirmation to the intuitive view that the evidence on which the results are based is reliable.

THE SECOND INTERVIEW: RESPONSES TO OPEN-ENDED QUESTIONS

Patient opinion of the hospital care was tested at the initial (discharge) interview by means of the patient service checklist. At the next interview, this was replaced by a series of seven open-ended questions designed to enable respondents to speak freely about their hospital experience and, particularly, about the nursing care received. This interview took place approximately 6 weeks after discharge when (it was hoped) the experience would still be fresh enough to recall, but the hospital remote enough not to inhibit free discussion. Spontaneous comments were sometimes recorded in another context and where possible these have been considered thematically and included in the analysis.

Although a total of 112 schedules were analysed, all of the questionnaires were not necessarily fully completed. As shown in Table 6.2, there was some attrition through reasons such as death or re-admittance to the ACU. As well, some of those that did participate in the second interview were incapable − or unwilling − to provide answers to all of the questions. As a result, not all of the following tables have a respondent total of 112.

The first two questions dealt with advice about convalescence.

Question 1

While you were in hospital, were you given any advice about what you should or shouldn't do during your convalescence?

Ninety-one replies were recorded out of a total of 112 schedules analysed (Table 7.1). Reasons for non-response included confusion, forgetfulness and dysphasia. One patient who was back in hospital at the time of the interview preferred not to answer.

Table 7.1 Advice about convalescence

Advice	Treatment	Control	Total
Yes	27 (42.2%)	11 (22.9%)	38 (33.9%)
No	26 (40.6%)	27 (56.3%)	53 (47.3%)
No information	11 (17.2%)	10 (29.8%)	21 (18.7%)
Total	64 (100%)	48 (100%)	112 (100%)

Table 7.2 Types of advice reported by control and treatment patients who answered yes to Question 1

Type of advice	Yes to Question 1	
	Treatment	Control
Exercise	12	3
Diet/smoking	3	3
Taking medicine	—	1
Hygiene	—	1
Kitchen/cooking	—	—
Miscellaneous	3	1
Cautionary	10	3
Encourage independence	4	2
Information irrelevent	2	2
Phone number given	2	—
Home visit	2	—

Question 2

Positive respondents were then asked to specify the type of advice they had received (Table 7.2). Six were unable to do so, because they either could not recall or could not explain what they had been told. One (treatment) implied that advice was not necessary, saying 'you should know what you should do' and one apparently misunderstood the question: 'Hospital staff did everything for me' (treatment).

Patients were not asked to distinguish between advice given by nurses and that given by other hospital staff, but it was sometimes stated that the advice had been given by physiotherapists.

Advice which was recalled by the remaining 30 patients in this group fell into two different categories: practical and general. Practical advice was given about specific areas of daily living, e.g. exercising, diet, smoking, taking medicine, hygiene and speech. Patients also remembered being advised to avoid heavy work such as lifting, to avoid going upstairs and not to bear weight on a leg for 3 months. Points from the home trials prior to discharge were remembered by two people (both treatment), e.g. loose rugs.

The other type of advice was more general, relating to returning to normal life at home. Sometimes the development of self confidence and independence was stressed: 'Help yourself'; 'Rely on yourself'; 'Look after yourself'; 'They said "can you do it?". I said, "yes"!' But conversely, others were cautioned against overactivity: 'Be careful'; 'Take things slowly/easy'; 'Go steady'; 'Don't overdo it'.

Two patients (both treatment) reported that they had been given the nurse's phone number to ring in case of need.

Numbers were similar between control and treatment patients for most categories of advice *except* advice of a general cautionary nature which was quoted by 13 treatment patients but only two in the control, and advice about exercising (including advice given by physiotherapists) which was recalled by 12 treatment patients and three controls.

Comments by those who replied 'no' to Question 1
Negative respondents to Question 1 should not have answered Question 2. However, 17 of the 53 in fact did so, sometimes in a way which suggested, e.g. 'Only the physiotherapist' [sic. gave advice] (control) or '[I was] told a bit about walking with a frame', (control). One person emphasised (treatment) that 'it was the GP gave exercises, *not* the hospital.' Another commented that much more advice and physiotherapy (treatment) had been offered after a previous stroke in 1972. It was not clear if this was due to the patient's increasing age or a change in the availability of health care.

The advice reported was similar to that for positive respondents to question 1, being either practical (including three or four

Table 7.3 Types of advice reported by control and treatment patients who answered 'no' to Question 1

Type of advice	No to Question 1 Treatment	Control
Exercise	—	3
Diet/smoking	—	1
Taking medicine	3	—
Hygiene	—	—
Kitchen/cooking	2	1
Miscellaneous	—	—
Cautionary	4	1
Encourage independence	2	1
Information irrelevent	—	1
Phone number given	—	—
Home visit	1	—

references to using the kitchen) covering exercise, advice on going upstairs, diet, medicine and rest, or generally cautionary (one control, four treatment); two patients again referred specifically to the home trial as the occasion when the advice was given. Perhaps it was remembered more easily from the home setting.

In summary, relatively few patients reported having been given advice but of those who did, more were from the treatment group (Table 7.3).

Questions 3 and 4

Patients were next asked *'Would you have liked more information or advice?'* and 88 replies were received to this question (three did not reply.) Question 4 asked them for specific details. Table 7.4 relates these to the answers given to Question 1.

Table 7.4 Response to Question 3 linked to Question 1

Response assessed as:	Treatment	Control	Total
Yes	4	2	6
No	22	7	29
No Response	1	2	3

Response assessed as:	Treatment	Control	Total
Yes	9	8	17
No	17	19	36
No Response	26	17	53

Response assessed as:	Treatment	Control	Total
Yes	13	10	23
No	39	26	65
No Response	1	2	3

Group A1
Only six of those who stated that they were given advice wanted more, but this group was important in that five out of the six (two control and three treatment) were expressing a psychological need, either for reassurance at a moment in life when the future

looked bleak, or at least for help in coping with life outside the
security of the hospital setting – 'To say how long I would be in
this state and how to cope when I got home' (control patient with
a fractured neck of femur). The advice this patient had actually
been given was to look after herself and take things easy. She
sought to excuse what might be taken as criticism of hospital staff
by saying: 'They were so busy. They had no time'. Four were
patients with a CVA (one control and three treatment) and they all
would have liked to have known about their prospects for
recovery, whereas the advice they had received was about diet
and exercise. It seems that help with practical problems was seen
by patients as less important than coming to terms emotionally
with possible long term disability (*cf*. Ahlsiö et al, 1984; Lawrence
and Christie, 1979).

Group A2
Group A2 consisted of those who had found the advice they had
been given adequate: 'They knew what you needed to be told'
(control) but one struck a positive note by saying: 'I would give
them 100% up there!' (treatment).

Group B1
Seventeen patients (eight control and nine treatment) who had
given a negative reply to Question 1 stated that they would have
liked information or advice prior to discharge. Again there was a
distinction between general advice on how to cope, e.g. 'I was not
told how much activity to undertake or whether to take things
slowly' (control patient with a CVA), and practical information
mainly to do with physical problems, e.g. 'How to manage my
leg'; 'How to get my hand moving'; 'How to walk on my own';
'About improving my eyesight'.

Seven patients (two control and five treatment), including some
of those just quoted, wanted more physiotherapy, but at least two
of these were in residential care and describing their current
situation, not advice received in hospital. Those and others like
them may have had unrealistic expectations regarding their
recovery.

More information was required by a few patients. The wife of a
heavily dependent patient with a stroke (control) commented that
she had to find things out for herself, e.g. about available
equipment, and would have benefitted from being given more

information. There seems to be no reason why such information should not be readily available.

Group B2
A surprisingly high proportion in both groups of those who replied (approximately 40%) had neither received advice or felt the need for any. At least half made no further comment and those who did were either 'quite satisfied' or took the view that no further help was possible. One patient in residential care commented that she was being looked after anyway (control).

Two interesting replies in this group touched on discharge arrangements. Both were made by patients with a CVA. The first, a widow (treatment), had two daughters and arrangements were made for her to be discharged to the one living nearby. Unfortunately, this arrangement broke down after a fortnight when the patient went back home barely able to cope alone. By the time of the second interview, she claimed that she had been worried all along about going to her daughter and it became clear that she got on better with the other daughter who lived further away. However, she was not at that stage prepared to move away to live with her. The family meanwhile felt 'all-at-sea', worried about their mother, but not knowing how to cope.

In the other case, the patient (control) was a married man discharged eventually to his own home. He expressed satisfaction with these arrangements which had been worked out not with his wife but by the social worker. He perceived this as being the social worker's role, but it did not occur to him that she had a role helping him to come to terms with his own disability and the 'vast change in personality' which he had experienced as a result of his stroke. This he described as 'a closely guarded secret' and 'not approved of in hospital'. It was only after returning home that he recognised it and had to try to cope with its results.

Both case histories emphasise the need for adequate preparation prior to discharge especially for stroke patients.

Question 5
What was good about the nursing your received in hospital? (Table 7.5)

Group A – positive
Patients' perceptions of what constituted 'good' nursing care focused mainly on human qualities rather than technical

efficiency. *Friendliness* was highly regarded, along with a homely/happy atmosphere on the ward. Nurses were appreciated as *loving/caring people* who were kind and cheerful. *Availability* and personal attention were also mentioned. 'Personal attention was very good. The nurses were always joking. They jollied you along'. One patient, perhaps more perceptively, appreciated the fact that 'They made you be independent' (treatment). 'They were good to me'; 'Lovely to me'; 'Nice to me', etc., were frequent comments.

Table 7.5 Response to Question 5

Response assessed as:	Treatment n	(%)	Control n	(%)	Total
A Positive	14	(22.2)	9	(19.5)	23
B Generally commendatory	32	(50.8)	19	(41.3)	51
C Neutral (no complaints)	6	(9.5)	7	(15.2)	13
D Non-committal or critical	3	(4.8)	3	(6.5)	6
No reply	8	(12.7)	8	(17.4)	16
Total	63		46		109

Group B – generally commendatory
These patients rated kindliness highly, along with friendliness, consideration and personal attention.

These comments differed only from Group A in being less specific, but in general the two overlap. Being talked to and not being hurried were each mentioned once with approval (both treatment). 'Are there any better people than nurses?' asked one patient, adding 'They do what you ask, as long as you are a patient patient. I didn't trouble them more than I could possibly help' (treatment).

Group C – neutral
These comments were either non-committal, e.g. 'No complaints'; 'Quite good'; 'I couldn't see any fault' or expressed certain reservations, especially about staff shortages – 'The nurses were very kind, but overworked'; 'They were very kind, but so limited because there were not enough of them' (both control).

One hundred and thirteen patients (or their relatives) said they did not need much nursing. In one of these cases (treatment), his wife had put the patient to bed every night and helped to feed him. Another asserted that 'The commode was all I needed' (treatment) and the third said 'Nurses were kind; I had nothing against them, but I didn't have much nursing' (control). One patient (control) said that it varied according to the staff on duty. He had reprimanded one nurse, but said that others were very good.

Group D – non-committal or critical
There were only three truly negative comments: 'I don't know that any was good, (they were) short of staff' (treatment).; 'I can't think of anything good, (I was) glad to get out' (control); 'It was awful. I was in a men's ward. I got used to the male nurse and preferred him, (control). The other three comments were wholly non-committal.

Question 6

What was not so good about the nursing you received in hospital? (Table 7.6)

Table 7.6 Response to Question 6

Response assessed as:	Treatment		Control		Total
	n	(%)	n	(%)	
A No complaint	39	(61.9)	15	(32.6)	54
B Non-specific criticism	2	(3.2)	5	(10.9)	7
C Specific complaint	10	(19.0)	10	(21.7)	22
No reply	12	(19.0)	10	(21.7)	22
Total	63	(100.0)	46	(100.0)	109

Nearly three-quarters of treatment group patients had no complaints, whereas over half the control group expressed criticism.

Group A – no complaints
Over half of all patients who replied had no complaints. Many of these replies were quite brief, e.g. 'No, nothing'; 'I don't think so'; 'No complaints'.

Others said more, for example, 'They were there if you wanted them'; 'I had everything I asked for'; 'I never felt ill-treated in any way'; 'Nothing — (they were) so very nice to me' (treatment patients).

'I didn't find any fault with them'; 'Nothing bad against them. Just asked them and they were there'; 'Anything I wanted I usually got it'; 'No, not to my way of thinking. [I was] in their care and had to abide by their ruling' (control patients).

Two in this group expressed the sentiment 'Home is best, but if you have to be in hospital it was alright'.

Group B/C
Any patients expressing dissatisfaction have been included in these groups, even when it was prefaced '[There was] nothing wrong, but ...'

The most common reasons for dissatisfaction were:
1. Staff shortage (five control and four treatment)
2. Connected problems were: waiting for service by nurses and being unable to attract their attention (especially when needing the commode) (five control and three treatment).

Other areas for complaint concerned:
1. Toileting (two control and two treatment).
2. Incompetence or roughness by nurses (four control and one treatment).
3. Rudeness or incompetence of non-nursing staff (one control and one treatment).
4. Embarrassment at being nursed by opposite sex (one control and one treatment).
5. Inattention/forgetfulness (by nurses) (one control and one treatment).
6. Food (two control).
7. Two patients (one control and one treatment) identified design faults causing discomfort. One in the shape of bedpans and one in the hardness of the beds!
8. One (control) patient complained that another patient had removed her possessions to his locker, implying lack of supervision by staff. One (treatment) patient had difficulty in identifying staff, because they did not wear uniform.
9. The wife of one patient with a stroke (treatment) thought that patients were put to bed too late at night both at the acute hospital, where she suggested the reason was that staff had

to be at reporting sessions with the change of shift at the time when many patients wanted to settle down for the night, and at the nursing unit, which she thought was rather understaffed at night.

10. One patient (treatment) felt she was 'in the wrong place'. She was a younger person with a fractured neck of femur and found that other more elderly and dependent patients claimed too much attention.

11. Two patients (both control) were not specific, saying 'It was too clinical.' and 'Sometimes, a very few.' (sic Nurses?).

Complaints about toileting

1. Usually this concerned either waiting for the commode to be brought or being left on the commode for a long time. In one case (control) the patient wet the bed because of the delay, but this was not due to staff shortages. She claimed that the nurses were chatting together and did not pay attention. One other patient thought that in cold weather she should have been allowed to use the commode instead of walking all the way to the toilet (treatment).

Technical incompetence

1. One incident happened when a student nurse gave the patient a shower: 'I took it as a joke, but she could have got into trouble' (control).

2. One high-dependency patient with a stroke had two complaints: the blind was not drawn for her against the sun, and her food was put in such a position that she could not (easily) feed and then it was removed too quickly (control).

3. One patient, with a stroke, was not washed thoroughly so that the soap was left caked on his skin, causing irritation. This he attributed to staff shortage: 'There were 16 men to wash between 6 and 8 am' (control).

4. One involved a leaking catheter. 'This hasn't happened again at home' (control).

5. One complained that her eyedrops were forgotten (treatment).

6. One complained that physiotherapists forced him to exercise and once he fell down (control).

The replies were next matched with replies to the previous question.

A. Of those with no complaints, all but six (four treatment and two control) patients had replied positively to Question 5. Three of these patients were dysphasic or forgetful.
B. (Non-specific criticism): three had replied positively to Question 5 and four were neutral or derogatory.
C. (Specific criticism): 18 had replied positively to Question 5, five had been neutral and three had been critical.

The three most explicitly critical patients in Question 5 were included in the specific complaints group in Question 6.

Question 7

Question 7 consisted of a series of open-ended sentences which were designed to elicit spontaneous comments mainly about the quality of nursing care (Table 7.7). Some difficulty was experienced in administering this part of the questionnaire, as many patients found it hard to understand that *they* were supposed to complete the sentences. The response rate was therefore relatively poor for this section, particularly under Question 7(c). However, when it worked, the method produced some heartfelt and also some amusing responses.

Table 7.7 Response to open-ended questions (Question 7)

Question	Useful information*	No relevant information	No reply	Total
7(a)	30	41	23	94
7(b)	61		34	95
7(c)	69		22	91
7(d)	56		37	93
7(e)	28	1	62†	91

*A reply which was relevant and meaningful.
†No reply includes the response 'nothing'.

Question 7(a): The most difficult thing to ask the nurse about was . . .
The interviewer first explained to the respondent what was required. Only a third completed this question in a meaningful and relevant way. Toileting was the problem mentioned most frequently as causing embarrassment (18 patients) especially

where staff were of the opposite sex to the patient (four). Forty one patients could not think of anything to say, others said they had experienced no difficulty because 'staff were broadminded'.

Question 7(b): As far as the nurses were concerned, I always knew . . .

In this section the largest group of answers expressed confidence in the *reliability* of nurses: e.g. 'I knew I could rely/depend on them' (several treatment and control); 'I knew they were there' (several treatment and control); 'I knew I'd be all right' (control); 'I knew I would get any attention needed' (control); 'I knew they'd come if I wanted' (treatment).

Associated with this were replies which stressed their *helpfulness:*. 'They were there to help' (control); 'That I would get done what I wanted' (treatment); and (even) 'That they would do as they were told!' (treatment).

Replies of this type often mentioned *human qualities* such as 'kind' and 'nice' and there were some embellishments: e.g. 'I knew them by their happy laugh' (control); 'They were well-dressed and clean' (treatment).

Kindness was seen to be important by five patients (one control and four treatment) and other replies supplied the same, e.g. 'I knew I would be well treated' (treatment).

Two patients thought the nurses were approachable: 'I could talk to them over anything' (treatment); 'If you asked any question, they would tell you' (treatment).

However, three patients *differentiated* between nurses: e.g. 'Some were fine, some were not' (treatment); 'Couldn't contact some – perhaps they were shy'; 'One nurse against another' (treatment). 'Some (were) distant and high, some were very nice' (control).

Three replies referred to *routine:* 'I knew what was coming next' (treatment). [Was this good or bad?]; 'I knew my turn would come' (control); 'I knew who to ask for what I wanted' (treatment).

However, one patient (treatment) *did not* know where they (the nurses) were and one had felt rushed: 'I knew when they wanted to hurry you up'.

The main points raised were therefore:

1. Reliability – associated with helpfulness – 38 replies (18 control and 20 treatment).

2.   Kind, nice, a sense of humour – 11 replies (3 control and 8 treatment).
3.   The importance of hospital routines and identifying personnel for patients' sense of security was emphasised by only a few patients.

Question 7(c): The nurses always . . .
This proved particularly hard for repondents to understand. Nevertheless there were similar categories to the previous section with a strong emphasis on *helpfulness, reliability* and *availability*.

Thirty four replied: 'Obliged/were attentive/helpful' (both groups); 'Answered your bell' (control); 'Were there when you wanted them' (one treatment and one control); 'Were at your right hand'(!) (treatment); 'Gave every attention' (treatment).

Eight patients (two control and six treatment) commented on the personal interest shown by nurses: 'Asked how I was' (control); 'Listened to me' (control); 'Reassured me' (treatment); 'Came to see if I was all right and had a word when they went by' (treatment); 'Praised you when you achieved something' (treatment – a stroke patient who recounted an incident at the dinner table).

Twenty-two commented on personal qualities, such as: cheerful, kind, patient, hardworking, polite, good (seven control and fifteen treatment).

Two remarked on nurse efficiency – that they tried to do their best: 'Did their job well' (control); and (from a former nurse!) 'Are in charge' (treatment).

Two control and three treatment replied 'remote' or 'in a hurry'.

On the other hand, several patients described nurses with these comments: 'They never had time enough' (control); 'She'd say, "I've only got two hands"' (treatment); 'Nobody had to do much for me' (treatment); 'Didn't have a lot to do with them except at night' (treatment); 'They answered my requests eventually' (control).

One patient replied: 'The nurses always brought things when you asked for them.' but added 'That's a lie' (control).

Question 7(d): If it hadn't been for the nurses, I would have . . .
Replies to this were sometimes quite jocular and ranged from actual survival to longer recovery time. Some form of dependency, physical or emotional, was the point most frequently made.

Survival: 12 said that they would not have survived, several in quite theatrical language: 'I would have shot myself' (treatment); 'Not lived through it' (control); 'Taken a gutfull of pills quickly' (control).

One patient stated matter-of-factly that there would be no hospital without the nurses (control).

Longer recovery: 10 patients (five control and five treatment) answered in such terms as; 'I would have taken longer to recover' (control); 'Not got on so well' (control); 'Still be in hospital now' (two treatment); 'Not been so well as I am now' (one control and one treatment).

Seven were quite non-committal (three control and four treatment): e.g. 'They treated me all right' (control); 'Rather have been at home' (treatment); and [bleakly] – 'Done without' (treatment).

The largest group answered in terms of dependency and inability to cope (five control and 11 treatment): 'Not known what to do' (treatment); 'They fed and looked after me' (treatment); 'Been in a mess, wouldn't I?' (control); and more colourfully: 'Been in a devil of a stew [they] were the only ones [I had] to rely on' (control); 'Been in a heck of a mess at times' (treatment); 'Smelt to high heaven' [patient added he could have answered the question in 1000 ways] (control); 'Grown more dependent and not been able to do as much for myself' (treatment).

Others mentioned emotional dependency (four control and one treatment): 'Felt miserable' (treatment); 'Been very lonely' (control); 'Been hopeless' (control); 'Been fed up and depressed' (control).

Question 7(e): Before going home, I would have liked it if . . .
Several quite distinct categories of responses were noted:

1. Feelings about home/discharge: some were so glad to go home there was nothing else they wanted (one control and two treatment) but others, though glad to go home, would have been willing to stay longer (five treatment).

2. Regret at leaving other patient/nurses: some expressed regret at not being able to say goodbye to other patients or staff (three treatment).

3. Desire to express gratitude tangibly: given the staff a present/thrown a party (one control and two treatment);

thanked all staff personally/given them something (one control and four treatment); taken one of the nurses with me (treatment).

4.   Complaints:
- one complaint concerned time of discharge (control);
- one complained that clothes were not aired (treatment);
- quite different were the replies (five control and one treatment) which expressed regret at the patient's own personal situation, e.g. I could have been able to walk/walk better (three control);
- one patient felt she had regressed since discharge because no physiotherapy was available in the nursing home where she was living (treatment); one said: 'I would have liked it if they had given me some advice on what to do and how long before I'd be able to get around normally' (control).

These replies highlight the problems of adjusting to a disability which were discussed earlier.

Question 8

Frankly, I would like to know what problems you have had since discharge, and if you have been able to cope with them.

Information was obtained on 105 patients, 13 of whom were in residential care. Some replies were very brief, and others detailed, the question sometimes opening up a discussion of problems which had been touched on earlier in the interview. These comments have been taken into account and also any points made by carers. One patient appeared to be upset by the question and refused to answer, possibly because she perceived her main problems to be with her family.

Table 7.8 Problems since discharge (non-residential care)

	Treatment		Control		Total
	n	(%)	n	(%)	
Group 1 (with problems)	36	(65.5)	21	(56.7)	57
Group 2 ('coping')	18	(32.7)	16	(43.2)	34
Refusal	1	(1.8)	—	(—)	1
Total	55		37		92

Responses were first divided into two main groups: those of patients who admitted to problems and those who did not. However, answers in the latter group were often qualified and it emerged that real problems had been encountered. The concept of 'coping' was often brought in (see Table 7.8).

Information was obtained for 13 patients in residential care, usually from staff, as detailed in Table 7.9.

Table 7.9 Problems since discharge (residential care)

	Treatment	Control	Total
Group 1 (with problems)	4	4	8
Group 2 ('coping')	1	3	4
Refusal	—	1	1
Total	5	8	13

Patients in residential care, whose physical needs are being met, may experience problems of a different type (e.g. restrictions on their independence and adaptation to communal living) to those living in their own homes. Replies have not, however, been analysed separately for those in residential care.

Group 1 (those admitting to problems)
Problems described by these 57 patients fell into five major groups:

1. Problems associated with *lack of mobility and dependency in general* caused by physical weakness or incapacity, including inability to climb stairs (12 control and 14 treatment).
2. *Health problems* included falls, speech problems, incontinence and medical set backs (8 control and 19 treatment).
3. *Environmental problems:* such as, housing, heating and including restrictions imposed because patient lived in an upstairs flat (4 control and 2 treatment).
4. *Psychological problems:* e.g. depression, frustration, anxiety, loss of confidence (10 control and 20 treatment).
5. *Dissatisfaction with/stress on carers* (2 control and 4 treatment).

The majority of problems were, predictably, associated either with poor health and lack of mobility or specific disability. Psychological problems assumed major importance for this group, especially depression, frustration, boredom, lack of concentration, anxiety and loss of confidence.

Group 2 (the 'coping' group)
There were 35 patients in this group, 12 of whom did not admit to any problems. Another 18 said they had no problems because help was available from family or other carers, including staff at residential homes.

The others admitted to problems but were able to cope and had similar difficulties to patients in Group 1. Twelve reported poor health or lack of mobility, but psychological problems were much less prominent than in Group 1 and it was perhaps patients' perceptions of problems more than the problems themselves which chiefly determined whether they were 'coping' or 'problem centred'.

THE THIRD INTERVIEW

The third interview took place 6 months after discharge from hospital and was shorter than the two previous interviews. It included only one open-ended question (similar to the last one in the second interview schedule). A total of 99 responses were received: death, readmittance to hospital or an inability to complete the questionnaire accounts for the difference between the number of respondents to interviews two and three.

I would like to know what problems you have had since the last two interviews and if you have been able to cope with them.

Not infrequently, there had already been some discussion of problems and difficulties in the course of the interview, e.g. when filling in the nursing dependency score. Sometimes, because the patient and researcher, not having met for some 4½ months, exchanged greetings and a formal enquiry might lead the respondent to launch into an account of his problems, even before the interview proper had started. This question might then be introduced by some remark such as, 'You have already told me about some of your difficulties. Are these your main problems or is there anything else?'. A summary of the previous discussion was then appropriate, in addition to the respondent's reply to the question as phrased.

As already shown in Chapter 6, the average life satisfaction score *increased* between the second and third interview, indicating that 6 months after discharge from hospital the study patients felt more positive about their situation and thus were more contented or, at least, had come to accept any residual disability or change in lifestyle. This average figure concealed of course a wide variation in life satisfaction, but suggested that respondents might report few or fewer problems than at the second interview.

Once again, it was the patient's perception of problems which was recorded; a reasonably objective outsider might have seen things differently. For example, the wife of an amputee (control), reported 'No special problems; he is able to get out in the wheelchair sitting in the sun', only mentioning in passing his ongoing medical problems and almost total dependence on her. Indeed one of the strongest impressions left with the interviewer was how frequently problems were understated or cheerfully accepted. 'There are many worse off than myself' may be a catch-phrase, but sounded poignant coming from a widower, living alone, suffering from Parkinsonism, and heavily dependent on health and social services to remain independent (treatment). The same philosophical attitude was expressed by a man (treatment) who spoke of 'accepting the situation and being thankful you are as well as you are'. This was a man who, at the second interview, had been depressed and disorientated at having to give up his own home when discharged to residential care.

The 99 schedules were analysed and replies were again sorted before being identified as control or treatment. The results are shown in Table 7.10. Of the 30 patients (12 control and 18 treatment) who reported 'no problems', 11 were living in residential care. Although the staff might disagree, the patients saw themselves as relieved of anxiety about their activity of daily living and most had adjusted to the dependent status. Of the other 19, all of whom were still living in their own homes, 5 at least showed some evidence of a mobility problem (e.g. one fractured neck of femur patient [control] who had not yet felt confident enough to go on a bus). Two respondents were uncommunicative: one man had become a recluse before hospitalisation, following the death of his wife; the other was a patient with a CVA (control)

Table 7.10 Number of patients reporting problems at 6/12 interview

| | Treatment | | Control | | Total |
	n	(%)	n	(%)	
No problem reported	18	(31.6)	12	(28.6)	30
Problem(s) reported	38	(66.6)	28	(66.7)	66
No reply	1	(1.8)	2	(4.7)	3
Total	57		42		99

who was dysphasic and was seen in hospital while his wife was on holiday. Problems undoubtedly were present in both cases.

No reply was received from three patients. One (treatment) was not seen, but her son (who was interviewed) made it clear that there were continuing health and psychological problems. The other two in this group (both control) were both in residential care and staff were interviewed by telephone in both cases.

It is probably true to say that only a few would echo the lady (treatment) who pronounced herself 'in perfect order!'. As might be expected in this age group, as with the 'coping' group at the second interview, continuing health problems were present in many cases, summed up by the man who was being visited regularly by the district nurse but who described himself as 'Not too bad; no particular problems. [I'm] about the same as before [I went] to hospital' (treatment).

Two-thirds of all patients interviewed 6 months after discharge reported problems and the proportion was similar for control and treatment groups.

The types of problems were divided into four main categories (and many patients of course, mentioned more than one type of problem). This was done before distinguishing a group or diagnosis. These categories were as follows:

1. *Mobility and related problems,* including the sense of isolation which reduced mobility can lead to, going upstairs and carrying things.
2. *Health problems* including re-admission to hospital, falling, pain, loss of use of limbs or of speech.
3. *Personal/practical problems.* This included finance and housing problems, as well as family difficulties associated with personal hygiene or toileting. This overlaps with health, but

was felt to be perceived more as a personal problem than a
health one.

4. *Psychological problems* – especially depression, frustration,
    aggression, obstructiveness, confusion, fear, lack of
    confidence, loneliness, and boredom.

The recovery prospects for elderly patients with a stroke is likely to
be very different to that of patients with a fractured neck of femur,
who can expect a virtually complete return to normal – certainly
this was the impression of the interviewer. The two diagnostic
groups were therefore considered separately in the analysis of this
question (Tables 7.11 and 7.12) although this had the disadvantage
that numbers were then too small to draw a distinction between
the control and treatment groups.

Table 7.11 Patients' response by diagnosis

Diagnosis	No problems	Problem(s) reported	Total
Fracture	18	22	40
CVA	10	41	51
Other	1	3	4

Table 7.12 Problems by diagnostic group and control/treatment

	Treatment		Control		Total
	n	(%)	*n*	(%)	
Fracture	10	(26.3)	12	(42.9)	22
CVA	25	(65.8)	16	(57.1)	41
Other	3	(7.9)	–	(–)	3
Total	38	(100)	38	(100)	66

In line with this expectation, it was found that 80% of cerebral
vascular accident patients reported problems compared to 55% of
fractured neck of femur patients.

Types of problems were then compared within these groups,
first for the number of patients and then the number of times
different types of problems reported.

In the fractured neck of femur group, *health related* and *psychological problems* were of equal importance (nine patients each).

Personal and practical problems were reported by seven patients. Three of these – all control patients – reported family problems.

Mobility problems were reported by six patients – two of these, both control patients, specifically mentioned a feeling of isolation. One of these, a woman who had been forced by her accident to retire from the job she enjoyed was missing the company it had given her. The other was a man whose life seemed to the interviewer to be restricted because he could no longer go out into town.

Similar results were obtained for the number of times different types of problems were reported.

Health-related problems were reported 13 times (including 3 reported re-admissions to hospital).

Psychological problems were reported 10 times.

Problems of restricted *mobility* were reported 8 times.

Personal/practical difficulties were reported 7 times. In the CVA group, 41 patients reported ongoing problems (16 control and 25 treatment).

Health problems were a major concern, with 30 patients in all reporting some health-related problem (including seven re-admissions). However, whereas 21 out of 25 treatment patients reported health problems, only 9 out of 16 control patients did so.

Psychological problems were reported by 18 patients, i.e. 50% of control patients who reported any problems had some psychological problem compared to 40% for the treatment group.

Mobility problems were reported by 13 patients (6 control and 7 treatment).

Personal/practical problems were reported by 14 patients (8 control and 6 treatment) – 50% of control patients with problems compared to 24% in the treatment group.

The pattern was similar for the number of times different problems were reported. *Health problems* were again the most frequent, with 38 reports (11 control and 27 treatment). Sixteen of these were reports from patients who had not fully recovered the use of limbs or of speech (5 control and 11 treatment).

Psychological problems – 22 reports (10 control and 12 treatment) with frustration and depression not unexpectedly being mentioned most frequently (6 control and 5 treatment).

Personal/practical problems – 18 reports (9 control and 9 treatment), e.g. worry about money or family problems (treatment patients), or about personal hygiene, use of commode or bathing (control).

Mobility problems – 15 reports, including 5 mentioning isolation. For 2 people (both treatment), failure (after 6 months) to fix handrails and make structural alterations meant that they could not leave the house unaided.

Patients in both diagnostic groups reported similar types of problems, but patients with a CVA reported more problems, especially general health problems and psychological problems. Patients with a CVA in both control and treatment groups were liable to experience depression, frustration, boredom and feelings of isolation.

A wife, who was coping with great ingenuity and determination with her husband's very severe physical dependence and loss of speech, said: 'Life is no fun anymore' (treatment). Another woman (control) put it differently: 'It's a bit long keeping indoors'.

Several found accepting their dependency the most depressing factor in their situation, because they had to watch helplessly whilst others did for them the tasks they used to do easily for others. 'Maybe I shall get more accustomed to this life', commented one man, as he described the frustration of watching his wife 'wrestling with' things he used to easily do for her (control). Another felt rejected by his son, who used to find him useful in running the house: 'There is so much I can't do now' (control). The attitude of relatives could also be hurtful when decisions appeared to be made without the patient's consultation: 'Because I am old and have had a stroke they think I can't know what I want for myself' (treatment). Another man (control) who was well able to verbalise his feelings, expressed bitterness at the attitude of former friends: 'Where do all your friends go?', a sentiment echoed by the lady quoted first in this paragraph who had found, when she took her husband out, that people he had known for 10 years would ignore his presence, addressing themselves exclusively to her.

8 Costs and cost-effectiveness

THE RESEARCH HYPOTHESIS

The research hypothesis in relation to the costs of care is that length of stay and/or cost per patient should be no longer/higher than for patients nursed on other wards. The length of stay has been examined in Chapter 6. In that chapter it was shown that the total length of stay in NHS care on average was longer for the treatment group than for the control group but that this difference was not statistically significant. In this chapter an attempt is made to compare the overall cost of care for the two groups.

COMPARISON OF COSTS BETWEEN THE NURSING UNIT AND ACUTE WARDS

The collection of financial data was very difficult as the health authority did not have data in a readily accessible form. Assistance was sought from the Health Authority's Treasurer's Department to establish the costs per bed, costs per case and costs per inpatient day. Accurate costing information for specific acute wards was not available and the Treasurer's Department was unable, despite a number of attempts, to generate information on costs per case or costs per inpatient day.

(Similar difficulties were encountered 18 months earlier in the pilot study, and estimated comparative costs were established by using a formula designed by the Health Authority's Treasurer's Department and District Planning Nurse. The introduction of new accounting systems in the near future is likely to remedy this limitation.)

The Treasurer's Department and District Planning Nurse were, however, able to produce comparative costings per bed, using recently collected financial information from two specific acute wards and the nursing unit.

The estimated cost per inpatient day is given in Table 8.1.

Table 8.1 Estimated cost per inpatient day for nursing unit

	Nursing Unit (£)
Estimated staff costs	130,800
Estimated non-staff costs	45,800
Total costs	176,600
Annual costs per bed (for 16 beds) (assuming 100% occupancy)	11,038
Mean cost per inpatient day	30.24

The estimated mean costs per inpatient day for acute hospitals is given in Table 8.2. These estimates have been obtained by averaging the cost figures obtained from the Health Authority for a 20 bed acute surgical ward and a 20 bed acute trauma ward.

Table 8.2 Estimated cost per inpatient day for acute hospitals

	Acute surgical (£)	Acute trauma (£)	Mean cost (£)
Estimated staff costs	168,400	190,640	179,520
Estimated non-staff costs	66,500	74,138	70,319
Total costs	234,900	264,778	249,839
Annual costs per bed (for 20 beds) (assuming 100% occupancy)	11,745	13,239	12,492
Mean cost per inpatient day	32.18	36.27	34.22

In Table 8.3 the cost per inpatient day is compared for the nursing unit and the acute wards. The acute hospital is £34.22 per day, while the nursing unit is £30.24 per day. Thus the nursing unit is shown to be £3.98 or 11.6% less per day than the acute ward.

Hence the nursing unit shows a lower cost per inpatient day compared with the acute hospital setting.

Table 8.3 Percentage saving per inpatient day

	Mean cost per inpatient day (£)
Acute hospital	34.22
Nursing Unit	30.24
Savings per inpatient day	3.98
Percentage saving per inpatient day	11.6%

There are a number of problems in estimating the costs per case for the treatment group and the control group. A major problem is that due to the large standard deviations in the number of days in acute care and in total NHS care there is some concern in using these estimates to determine total cost per case.

Table 6.7 from Chapter 6 is reproduced in this chapter as Table 8.4.

Table 8.4 Length of hospital stay by hospital and group

Hospital	Treatment group (n = 80) Mean (S.D.)		Control group (n = 63) Mean (S.D.)	
ACU	10.8	(9.2)	33.7	(29.0)
Nursing unit	36.6	(25.0)	NA	
Community hospital (n = 16)	NA		35.9	(30.6)
Total number of days	47.2	(27.5)	42.9	(32.8)

Another problem is that there was no cost data available for the Community Hospital. Although only 16 of the control group patients went to the Community Hospital they had a mean stay of 35.9 days and it is necessary to have costings for this component of the stay. The 35.9 days for 16 patients is only 9.2 days on average over the 63 patients in the control group.

One possible option is to assume that the costs of the community hospital were similar to the nursing unit. These results are shown in Table 8.5. Based on this assumption the cost per case is similar for both the treatment and the control group.

Table 8.5   Cost per case

	Number of days	Cost per bed (£)	Total cost (£)
Treatment group			
Acute stay	10.8	34.22	369.58
Nursing unit	36.6	30.24	1106.78
Cost per case for treatment group			1476.36
Control group			
Acute stay	33.7	34.22	1153.21
Community hospital	9.2	30.24	278.21
Cost per case for control group			1431.42

CONCLUSION

The overall conclusion is that the cost per inpatient day is less in the nursing unit compared with the acute setting by £3.98 per day or 11.6%. However, when this cost data is incorporated with the length of stay data from Chapter 6, the overall cost of care is slightly higher for the treatment group compared with the control group. Given the nature of the length of stay data, the findings on overall cost of care are not conclusive.

9 | Discussion

SAMPLE

The sample proved to be homogeneous between control and treatment groups in terms of age, sex and living situation before admission to hospital. In addition, there were no significant differences in the CAPE scores for the total sample (before deaths in hospital).

MORTALITY (DEATH IN HOSPITAL BEFORE INITIAL DISCHARGE)

A highly significant difference was found, with control group patients being three times more likely to die in hospital than treatment group patients. Admittedly, in the patients in a CVA group, which accounted for most of these deaths, higher CAPE scores were found, but as previously discussed, this was caused by higher scores for only two items which would not seem likely in themselves to be indicators of poor prognosis. Mortality rates were not a part of the research hypothesis and the finding was surprising and remains unexplained.

LENGTH OF STAY

Patients randomised to the treatment group were transferred to the nursing unit as soon as possible after acceptance into the study (see Chapter 5) so that it was not unexpected that length of stay in acute care would be lower than for the control group. Results show that control group patients spent on average three times as long in acute care as treatment patients. Overall, however, average length of stay was slightly longer for treatment group patients, but this difference was not significant and does not negate the hypothesis that length of stay in NHS care would be no more for treatment group patients than for those in the control group.

The reasons why patients transferred to the nursing unit should have had longer stays are speculative but may be linked to the lower dependency scores achieved by this group on discharge. Adequate preparation for discharge, with the patient fully involved in decision making wherever possible was part of the philosophy of the unit. This might result in a marginally longer average stay, but a more satisfactory placement on discharge. However, no data was collected about the success of living arrangements after discharge and no conclusions can be drawn about this.

The effect of diagnosis may also be important. The average stay at the nursing unit was longer for patients who had sustained a fracture of the neck of the femur but shorter for patients with a CVA (see Chapter 6, Table 6.9) than for the control group. The average length of stay for patients who had had amputations was 62.3 days for those in the treatment group, compared to 41.7 days in the control group; but the numbers involved were too small to draw conclusions.

The question of relative costs has been discussed in Chapter 8. Despite the slightly longer average stay recorded at the nursing unit, it is doubtful whether average total cost in the nursing unit would be higher than for patients nursed in acute care beds and community hospitals.

RE-ADMISSIONS

No reliable method of ensuring that all re-admissions of patients in the sample were evaluated was built into the study. It was, therefore, not possible to collect data consistently enough to support or reject the hypothesis.

QUALITY OF CARE

The measure used to assess quality of nursing care was the nursing audit score and the assumption was made that this would be valid. The results were significantly better for the treatment group with nearly all scores in the 'excellent' range, whereas the majority of control patients had 'good' or satisfactory' scores.

Scores were also *consistently* higher for the treatment group to a significant degree. Therefore the quality of nursing care as measured by the nursing audit score was not merely no worse at the nursing unit than that provided by other wards, but was found to be more satisfactory and consistently so, thus supporting the research hypothesis.

PATIENT SERVICE CHECK LIST

Another indirect measure of quality of care was the patient's assessment, as provided by the patient service check list. Although in the interviews a tendency to give what was thought to be the 'right' answer had been suspected, in the analysis it was shown that treatment group patients were significantly more satisfied with the nursing care they had received, using this check list, than those in the control group, thus confirming the third research hypothesis (see Chapter 6, Table 6.10)

Remarks made by patients at the interview 6 weeks after discharge tended to support this conclusion. When asked what was good about the nursing received in hospital, 83% of the treatment patients, compared to 73% of control patients, gave replies which were graded as 'positive' or 'generally commendatory'. When asked to specify anything about the nursing which was 'not so good', although less than half of those who replied could do so, three-quarters of the the treatment group had no complaints in comparison with just under half of the control patients.

NURSING DEPENDENCY SCORES

Nursing dependency on discharge was found to be significantly different for the two groups, with treatment group patients achieving significantly more independence in the activities of daily living than control patients.

Table 6.13 shows scores for activities requiring human assistance. This result does not merely support the hypothesis that care in the nursing unit would result in independence levels on discharge no lower than those achieved in other wards, but shows that on average, a better result was achieved than for control group patients. Possible reasons for this were discussed above, under Length of Stay. The fact that differences between the two groups were reduced by the time of the later interviews tends to confirm that it was the input from the nursing unit motivating patients towards self-care and achieving maximum possible independence that proved effective. Control group patients remained marginally more dependent 6 weeks and 6 months after discharge. Although these differences were not statistically significant, they suggested that when higher independence levels can be achieved in hospital, the improvement can be maintained after discharge.

LIFE SATISFACTION SCORES

Satisfaction with life in general was measured at each interview and the results showed no significant differences either between control and treatment groups or between diagnostic groups. This supported the hypothesis that levels of satisfaction with life in general would be no lower for patients discharged from the nursing unit than for those discharged from other wards.

The fact that there was no measurable difference in satisfaction with life between diagnostic groups is surprising. Several studies have shown the catastrophic effects on social satisfaction which patients with a stroke often experience. The severe stroke patients in this study faced fundamental changes in the quality of life and expectations for the future, and in some cases the interviewer witnessed the process of adjustment which had to be made.

The fact that these problems were not reflected in lower life satisfaction scores among patients with a CVA may be partly due to the inability to gain data caused by the difficulty of administering the Life Satisfaction index schedule to dysphasic patients in this group.

Another interesting point was the drop in life satisfaction scores between the first and second interviews. Six weeks after discharge, the problems of coping with life when some degree of disability was present were reflected in the scores; after 6 months, scores improved again, although still not to the level of the first interview. Improvement in health or adjustment to handicap had by this time taken place for the survivors (see Table 6.13).

Qualitative data regarding problems after discharge may appropriately be considered at this point. At the second interview, 6 weeks after discharge, 65% of treatment patients admitted to problems compared to 57% of control patients and similar results were obtained after 6 months. Yet there was no significant difference in life satisfaction scores between the two groups at either interview.

Patients who experienced care in the nursing unit were encouraged to verbalise their problems and were not discouraged from expressing negative feelings; this openness may have helped patients to cope with ongoing problems whilst still maintaining a reasonable level of life satisfaction. It also allowed them to complain more freely at interviews.

In general, results from the quantitative data analysis were more consistent across the board for treatment patients than for the control group. The standard deviation in all areas of quantitative measurement was notably lower for treatment patients, a group who had all experienced care in one nursing unit with a cohesive philosophy underpinning the delivery of nursing care; whereas control patients had been nursed in various wards in different hospitals. This may partially account for the difference but is hardly adequate as a complete explanation of such a striking result. No other factor provides a more satisfactory explanation than the possible effect of exposure to the therapeutic style of nursing care practiced in the nursing unit.

Qualitative data inevitably yields less rigorous results than data which is amenable to statistical analysis. Nevertheless it contributes to the total picture by adding depth and richness to the bare outline provided by the quantifiable data.

This group of elderly hospitalised patients emerged as generally tolerant, usually uncomplaining and reluctant to criticise their experience of health care generally and of nursing in particular. They valued highly personal qualities of kindness, friendliness, etc., in nurses, rather than technical skills, but tended not to remember much about the advice they had been given except in very general terms. Nurses were perceived as very busy people and specific criticisms of staff shortages was made by patients in both groups.

Treatment group patients were almost twice as likely as control group patients to remember being given advice in hospital about their convalescence (42% treatment, 23% control); specifically, advice on 'taking care' and taking exercise was reported by 20% in the treatment group but only 5% in the control group. They were less likely to be critical of the nursing care they had received; only 32% of treatment patients compared to 58% of the control group made general or specific complaints. They were, however, more likely to admit to problems 6 weeks after discharge (65% treatment, 33% control), but after 6 months this difference was less apparent. Problems were similar for both groups; health and mobility problems, psychological problems and miscellaneous personal, practical and financial problems were reported and miscellaneous personal, practical and financial problems were reported at second and third interviews by both control and treatment group patients. At the 6 month interview, in the group of patients with cerebral vascular accident, health problems were particularly prominent for treatment group patients, but a higher proportion of control patients in this sub-group reported psychological problems.

A small minority of younger treatment group patients had experienced boredom and depression at the nursing unit, complaining of lack of stimulus because of the age and dependency of fellow patients and lack of recreational facilities. Some who complained that the unit seemed understaffed could have been confused by the absence of uniformed staff and may have failed to appreciate the role in their care of ward orderlies and associate nurses.

More typically, however, patients who had experienced care at the nursing unit were complimentary, expressing cordial feelings of appreciation at the 'homely', 'family' atmosphere. 'Although I was ill', said one, 'I quite enjoyed it'. Similar sentiments were noted in the control group from three patients who had been nursed at one community hospital.

10 Conclusions and Recommendations

CONCLUSIONS

In summary, the results have shown that in a homogeneous sample of elderly patients, differences between control and treatment group patients have emerged which, it is purported, are the effect of the operation of the dependent variable, i.e. therapeutic nursing care at the nursing unit.

Four of the study hypotheses were supported, and the data strongly suggests that the nursing unit was successful in promoting recovery and increasing quality. In addition, there was evidence to show that costs *per day* in the nursing unit were significantly lower, although the evidence on cost *per case* was inconclusive.

The research hypotheses stated:

1. *That care in the nursing unit will be no worse than provided by other wards.*

   This was supported by nursing audit scores, and in fact quality of care as judged by these scores was found to be significantly higher, and more consistently so, in the nursing unit than in other wards.

2. *That care in the nursing unit will result in an independence level no lower than that achieved in other wards.*

   This was supported by the nursing dependency scores. Not only were these scores lower than those of patients cared for in other hospital wards, they were significantly so in patients who were cared for in the nursing unit, when they were discharged from hospital.

3.   *That patients discharged from the nursing unit will be no less satisfied with the nursing care received than patients in other wards.*

This was supported by the patient service checklist scores and the qualitative data obtained. Indeed, the patient service checklist scores were significantly higher in patients who were cared for in the nursing unit, there were fewer complaints about care in nursing unit patients 6 weeks after discharge, than in patients who were in the control group. Satisfaction with care was therefore higher in nursing unit patients.

4.   *That patients discharged from the nursing unit will have a level of satisfaction with life in general no lower than that of patients discharged from other wards.*

This was supported by life satisfaction scores, which were not significantly different between control and treatment groups.

5.   *That re-admission rates for patients discharged from the nursing unit will be no higher than those for patients discharged from other wards.*

This hypothesis could not be tested because of irresolvable problems in collecting this data.

6.   *That length of stay and/or cost per patient should no longer/higher than for patients nursed on other wards.*

This was supported by a significantly shorter average stay in the acute hospital for treatment group patients. However, the total length of stay in an NHS bed was higher for the treatment group than the control group but the difference was not significant. Although the cost per day was lower for the nursing unit the data on the cost per case was inconclusive.

Thus four of the six hypotheses were supported by the research findings, one hypothesis could neither be supported nor refuted because of lack of data and the findings for the final hypothesis were not conclusive.

In addition, significantly less treatment group patients died in hospital; significantly more were discharged to their own homes; and the results of the quantitative data were more consistent for treatment group patients with smaller standard deviations for most factors of analysis.

The findings therefore strongly indicate that nursing-led care has a positive effect on recovery, quality, satisfaction and mortality, which supports the study assumption that nursing in itself is a therapeutic force.

Contemporary health-care planners and policy makers explicitly and consistently urge for higher quality, better outcomes and lower costs. This study clearly demonstrates that nursing beds can achieve all three objectives.

RECOMMENDATIONS

Such results identify the need to maintain the experimental unit, and to replicate it in other areas of the NHS. The findings of this study clearly demonstrate the quantitative and qualitative benefits of providing therapeutic nursing in a designated nursing unit where nursing is the primary therapy, and nurses are the chief therapists. Nurses have been urged for many years to evaluate their effectiveness in patient care, and to demonstrate this with empirical data. Despite the enormous difficulty in producing such data in a field which is surrounded by extraneous variables, this study has generated data with very strongly identified trends. The need for the continuation and expansion of the independent variable in the study, i.e. the nursing unit, is indisputable in the light of the results. It is hoped that this will lead to an overall improvement in the service, both to the consumer, and to the organisation in the terms of cost effectiveness.

In view of the findings, it is recommended that:

1.   The experimental unit established for the study be maintained and strengthened in its existing form, and that its use by acute specialities be encouraged.

2.   That the findings of this study be disseminated widely, particularly to politicians, nursing and medical leaders, and health service leaders and planners.

3.   That further nursing units be established within the NHS, and further evaluation of their role and effectiveness be conducted.

4.   That the therapeutic effects of nursing on patients be seriously studied within the health care system.

5.   That further innovation within nursing be given more encouragement and financial support by governmental nursing departments.

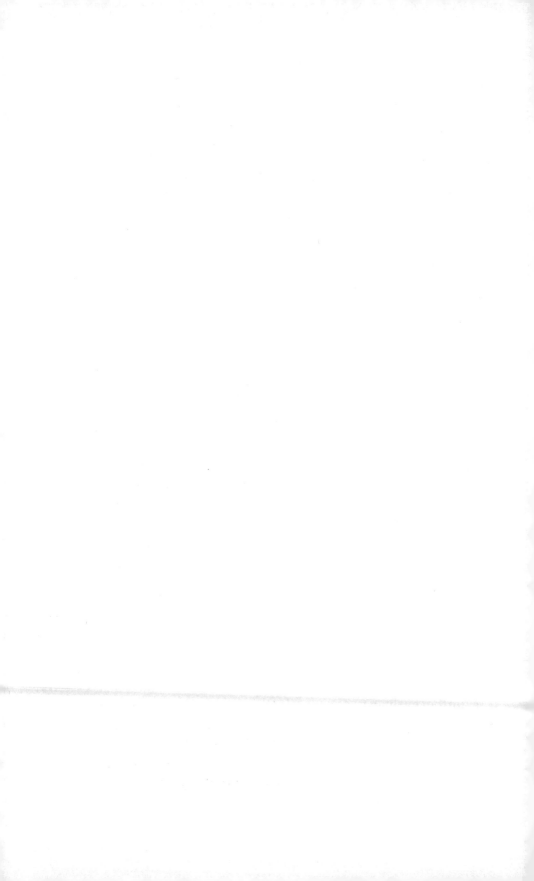

Appendix:
Forms used for survey

CODE NO: ☐☐☐
                                                                            1 2 3

SEX: Male = 1   ☐ 4
                              Female = 2

AGE: ☐☐☐
                                                                            5 6 7

DIAGNOSIS: (See diagnostic code list)   ☐ 8

SOURCE OF REFERRAL: 1 = Consultant geriatric firm   ☐ 9
                              2 = Ward Sister
                              3 = Houseman
                              4 = Consultant
                              5 = G.P.
                              6 = Liason Nurse
                              7 = Other

DAYS IN UNIT: ☐☐☐
                                                                            10 11 12

DISCHARGE TO: 1 = Own Home   ☐ 13
                              2 = Part III
                              3 = Community Hospital
                              4 = Acute Hospital
                              5 = Other (specify)

NURSE: 1 =   ☐ 14
                              2 =
                              3 =
                              4 =
                              5 =

UNIT DOCTOR: 1 =   ☐ 15
                              2 =
                              3 =

NURSING AUDIT SCORES: Function 1   ☐ 16
                                2   ☐ 17
                                3   ☐ 18
                                4   ☐ 19
                                5   ☐ 20
                                6   ☐ 21
                                7   ☐ 22
                       TOTAL   ☐ 23

BASIC BIOGRAPHIC SCHEDULE

INFORMATION TO BE TAKEN FROM PATIENT'S NOTES

INITIAL PATIENT HISTORY

PATIENTS NAME   _____   □ 1

INTERVIEWER NO.
i.e. 1, 2, 3 or 4   _____

DATE   _____

HOSPITAL NO.   _____   □□□
                                                              2 3 4

PATIENT'S CODE NO.   _____

MENSTRUAL STATUS BEFORE OP.
                       Menstruating   1   5
                       Menopausal   2
                       Post menopausal   3
                       Non applicable   4

DATE OF BIRTH   _____   6 □□7
                                                         8 □□9
                                                        □□□□
                                                     10 11 12 13

NUMBER OF CHILDREN   _____   □ 14

| SEX: | Male = 1 | |
| | Female = 2 | ☐ 15 |

HOME TEL NO: _____

DATE OF FRACTURE: _____

| DIAGNOSIS: | See codes 0–9 | ☐ 16 |

DATE OF OPERATION: _____

| OPERATION: | See codes 0–9 | ☐ 17 |

| CONSULTANT: | See codes 0–9 | ☐ 18 |

POST OP ANALGESIA: _____

| POST OP RECOVERY | Uneventful = 1 | |
| | Complication = 2 | ☐ 19 |

| INTRA-VENOUS THERAPY | Yes = 1 | ☐ 20 |
| | No = 2 | |

| WHEN MOBILISED | In days _____ | ☐ 21 |

| HISTORY OF POST-OP CONFUSION | Yes = 1 | ☐ 22 |
| | No = 2 | |

| GROUP: | Control 1 = 1 | |
| | Exp. = 2 | ☐ 23 |

INITIAL PATIENT HISTORY

NAME
_____ , I would like to ask you some questions
about yourself, your family and your social activities. To begin with:

1. At the present time are you . . . .

MARRIED	1
WIDOWED	2
DIVORCED	3
SEPARATED	4
NEVER MARRIED	5
CO-HABITING	6
NO INFORMATION	7

☐ 24

2. Where were you living before you came to this hospital?
   Address: _____
   _____

3. What are the names of the other persons who lived with you at that
   address, how old are they, and how are they related to you?

NAME	RELATIONSHIP	AGE

☐ 25
☐ 26
☐ 27

(Code: (0)=alone (1)=spouse (2)=child (3)=other relative or friend)

4. Of those you have just mentioned or anyone else not living with you
   which one person:

   a. Do you know best?   _____
   b. Spends the most time with you
      at home?   _____
   c. Will spend the most time with
      you after you leave hospital?   _____

5. What type of residence did you live in before you were hospitalised?

HOUSE	1
BUNGALOW	2
FLAT	3
WARDEN CONTROLLED	4
PART III ACCOMM.	5
OTHER	6
NO INFORMATION	7

☐ 28

6. Does your residence have? ...

STAIRS	1
NO STAIRS	2

☐ 29

INSIDE TOILET	3
OUTSIDE TOILET	4

☐ 30

CENTRAL HEATING	5
COAL/ELECTRIC FIRE	6
NO HEATING	7

☐ 31

7. Do you have to climb stairs to?   Yes = 1, No = 0

ENTER YOUR RESIDENCE	
GO TO TOILET	
GO TO BED	

☐ 32
☐ 33
☐ 34

8. Were you employed at the time you were hospitalised

YES	1
NO	2

☐ 35

9. When were you last employed?

LESS THAN A YEAR AGO	1
1–4 YEARS AGO	2
5 OR MORE YEARS AGO	3
NEVER WORKED	4
NO INFORMATION	

☐ 36

10. What type of work did you do?
    (this includes running your home) _____

11. Do you intend to return to work Yes = 1, No = 2

☐ 37

YES	
NO	

12. What is the highest grade you completed in school?

SECONDARY SCHOOL	1
GRAMMAR SCHOOL	2
COLLEGE/UNIV	3
NO INFORMATION	

☐ 38

Nursing Dependency Index

Patient Code Number ☐☐☐☐   Date of Visit ☐☐☐☐☐☐   Number of Visit ☐☐

Day Base ....   Interval since last visit (in days) ☐☐

Activity* Important note: Only score ONE performance per activity						
*See Definition Sheet Performance of A.D.L. activity	Independent	Independent with aids	Required Assistance of no more than 1 person	Requires Assistance of no more than 2 persons	Bedfast	Activity Score
	Score 1 /activity	Score 2 /activity	Score 3 /activity	Score 4 /activity	Score 5 /activity	
1. Bed						
2. Dressing						
3. Walking						
4. Toileting						
5. Provision of meal						
6. Feeding						
7. Control of environment						
8. Washing and grooming						
9. Bathing or shower						
10. Chair						
11. Wheelchair						
12. Bladder function						
13. Bowel function						
14. Medication						
15. Treatment						
16. Management of household						
17. Emotional health						
18. Sleep						
19. Time up during day						
PERFORMANCE SCORE						

Nursing Dependency Index: Professional Sources of Assistance

Patient Code Number ☐☐☐☐   Number of visit ☐☐

	GP	DNS	HV	MSW	ASW	HHS	MOW	VA	CH		DH	OT	PT	Res	Oth	Act. Sc.
Professional Source of Assistance																
1. Bed																
2. Dressing																
3. Walking																
4. Toileting																
5. Provision of meal																
6. Feeding																
7. Control of Environment																
8. Washing and grooming																
9. Bathing or shower																
10. Chair																
11. Wheelchair																
12. Bladder Function																
13. Bowel Function																
14. Medication																
15. Treatment																
16. Management of household																
17. Emotional health																
18. Sleep																
19. Time up during day																
Professional Sources Score																

Activities of Living Assessment

Nursing Dependency Score	39 ☐ ☐ 40
Total dependency requiring human assistance	41 ☐ ☐ 42
Bed	☐ 43
Dressings	☐ 44
Mobility	☐ 45
Hygiene	☐ 46
Preparation – hot drink, simple snack	☐ 47
Feeding	☐ 48
Environment	☐ 49
Washing and grooming	☐ 50
Bathing or shower	☐ 51
Chair	☐ 52
Wheelchair	☐ 53
Bladder Function	☐ 54
Bowel Function	☐ 55
Medication	☐ 56
Treatment	☐ 57
Management of household	☐ 58
Emotional Health	☐ 59
Sleep	☐ 60
Time up during day	☐ 61

Life Satisfaction Profile

How often do you do the following activities?
(See list below for possible answers)

1. Reading books, newspapers or magazines ....   ☐ 62

2. Taking walks ....   ☐ 63

3. Sewing, knitting or crocheting ....   ☐ 64

4. Watching TV or listening to the Radio ....   ☐ 65

5. Visiting friends or relatives at their home ....   ☐ 66

6. Making dinner for friends or relatives ....   ☐ 67

7. Attending cinema, theatre or sporting events ....   ☐ 68

8. Social games (Chess, Dominoes, Cards, Bingo) ....   ☐ 69

9. Fishing, hunting, golf, bowling or other sports ....   ☐ 70

10. Playing a musical instrument ....   ☐ 71

11. Hobbies (Stamp collecting, model making, dressmaking etc) ......   ☐ 72

	Code		*Code*		*Code*
EVERY DAY	6	ONCE A WEEK	4	ONCE A MONTH	2
2 OR 3 TIMES		ABOUT TWICE		A COUPLE OF	
A WEEK	5	A MONTH	3	TIMES A YEAR	1
				NEVER	0
				NO INFORMATION	X

12. Do you belong to any clubs or organisations which hold regular meetings?

YES	1
NO	2
NO INFO.	X

☐ 73

13. What are these organisations, and how often do they meet? (SEE LIST)

14. How often did you attend meetings? (see list)

....

15. Were you an officer or have any special responsibilities such as chairman or member of a committee? (see list)

....

16. About how much time all together (per week or per month) did you devote to your organisation, including all meetings, functions and other work done?

....

List

Organisation	Frequency of meetings	Time spent	How often patient attended	Positions held and duties

☐ 74
☐ 75
☐ 76
☐ 77

1	2	3
Agree	Disagree	Undecided

Check boxes from right to left within a diagonal line with an X score one point.

17. As I grow older, things seem better than I thought they would be. | 1 | 2 | 3 | ☐ 78

18. I have had more chances in life than most of the people I know. | 1 | 2 | 3 | ☐ 79

19. This is the dreariest time of my life. | 1 | 2 | 3 | ☐ 80

20. I am just as happy now as when I was younger. | 1 | 2 | 3 | ☐ 81

21. My life could be happier than it is now. | 1 | 2 | 3 | ☐ 82

22. These are the best years of my life. | 1 | 2 | 3 | ☐ 83

23. Most of the things I do are boring or monotonous. | 1 | 2 | 3 | ☐ 84

24. I expect some interesting and pleasant things to happen to me in the future. | 1 | 2 | 3 | □ 85

25. The things I do today are as interesting to me as they ever were. | 1 | 2 | 3 | □ 86

26. I feel old and somewhat tired. | 1 | 2 | 3 | □ 87

27. As I look back on my life I am fairly well satisfied. | 1 | 2 | 3 | □ 88

28. I would not change my past even if I could. | 1 | 2 | 3 | □ 89

29. I like to take an interest in my appearance. | 1 | 2 | 3 | □ 90

30. I have made plans for things I'll be doing in a month or a year from now. | 1 | 2 | 3 | □ 91

31. When I think back over my life, I didn't get most of the important things I wanted. | 1 | 2 | 3 | □ 92

32. Compared to other people, I get down in the dumps too often. | 1 | 2 | 3 | □ 93

33. I've got pretty much what I expected out of life. | 1 | 2 | 3 | □ 94

34. In spite of what people say, the life of the average person is getting worse not better. | 1 | 2 | 3 | □ 95

Total Score LSI – A Boxes with an X score one point.

96 97
□   □

Patient Service Check List (Discharge)

NAME: _____I am pleased that you are now able to leave hospital, before you go could I please ask some questions about your stay in hospital?

	TRUE	NOT TRUE	NOT APPLICABLE	
35. The radio or TV was noisy.	2	1	X	☐ 98
36. My bed bath was not given to me when I wanted it.	2	1	X	☐ 99
37. The nurse was usually in a hurry.	2	1	X	☐ 100
38. Couldn't get anything from nurse for pain.	2	1	X	☐ 101
39. The nurse was prompt in answering my call.	2	1	X	☐ 102
40. Food trays were removed as soon as I was finished.	2	1	X	☐ 103
41. Thermometer left in too long.	2	1	X	☐ 104
42. Didn't see nurse often enough.	2	1	X	☐ 105
43. My bedpan or commode was removed promptly.	2	1	X	☐ 106
44. My food was served at the right termperature.	2	1	X	☐ 107
45. Nurse or assistants left me with clean towels.	2	1	X	☐ 108
46. My meals were served as I had ordered.	2	1	X	☐ 109
47. Drinking water was changed regularly.	2	1	X	☐ 110
48. Other patients made disturbing noises.	2	1	X	☐ 111
49. Nurse left before I could ask her questions.	2	1	X	☐ 112
50. Had to wait too long for a bedpan.	2	1	X	☐ 113
51. The nurses offered to stay with me when I was first allowed up.	2	1	X	☐ 114
52. The nurses fed me when I needed help.	2	1	X	☐ 115
53. My room was comfortable to sleep in.	2	1	X	☐ 116
54. I was not propped up, making it hard to enjoy my meal.	2	1	X	☐ 117

	TRUE	NOT TRUE	NOT APPLICABLE	
55. The nurses never told me how they were going to care for me.	2	1	X	☐ 118
56. The nurses let me do things at my own speed.	2	1	X	☐ 119
57. The nurses offered to bathe me when I needed help.	2	1	X	☐ 120
58. Light was too bright when I tried to sleep.	2	1	X	☐ 121
59. The hallways near my room were fairly quiet.	2	1	X	☐ 122
60. Nurses seemed very interested in me.	2	1	X	☐ 123
61. Bathroom was not clean.	2	1	X	☐ 124
62. My bath, meal or rest period was interrupted by treatment.	2	1	X	☐ 125
63. If I felt bad, I was not asked to do anything I didn't want to do.	2	1	X	☐ 126
64. I was awakened to have my temperature taken.	2	1	X	☐ 127
65. Was not served drinks after I requested them.	2	1	X	☐ 128
66. In general, my room was neat and tidy.	2	1	X	☐ 129
67. The nurses wouldn't tell me what was wrong with me.	2	1	X	☐ 130
68. My food was cold when served.	2	1	X	☐ 131
69. The nurses were very nice to me.	2	1	X	☐ 132
70. The nurses were with me fairly often.	2	1	X	☐ 133
71. Bed was not changed often enough.	2	1	X	☐ 134
72. The patients near me were fairly quiet.	2	1	X	☐ 135
73. Nurse did not wash and rub my back well.	2	1	X	☐ 136
74. The nurse was not prompt in answering my call.	2	1	X	☐ 137
75. Air in my room was always fresh.	2	1	X	☐ 138
76. I didn't get medicine when I requested it.	2	1	X	☐ 139
77. The nurses take their time with me.	2	1	X	☐ 140

	TRUE	NOT TRUE	NOT APPLICABLE	
78. My bandage or dressing was too tight.	2	1	X	☐ 141
79. Bedpan was brought to me promptly.	2	1	X	☐ 142
80. I was given a wheelchair when I asked for one.	2	1	X	☐ 143

ADDITIONAL COMMENTS:

81. No. of days in acute hospital				144/145/146
82. No. of days in a community hospital				147/148/149
83. No. of days in a nursing unit				150/151/152

84. Discharged to: home = 1, Part III = 2
    N.H.S. hosp = 3, Private home = 4   153
    Others = 5

Nursing Dependency Index

Patient Code Number ☐☐☐☐   Date of Visit ☐☐☐☐☐☐   Number of Visit ☐☐

Day Base . . . .   Interval since last visit (in days) ☐☐

Activity* Important note: Only score ONE performance per activity						
*See Definition Sheet Performance of A.D.L. activity	Independent	Independent with aids	Required Assistance of no more than 1 person	Requires Assistance of no more than 2 persons	Bedfast	Activity Score
1. Bed	Score 1 /activity	Score 2 /activity	Score 3 /activity	Score 4 /activity	Score 5 /activity	
2. Dressing						
3. Walking						
4. Toileting						
5. Provision of meal						
6. Feeding						
7. Control of environment						
8. Washing and grooming						
9. Bathing or shower						
10. Chair						
11. Wheelchair						
12. Bladder function						
13. Bowel function						
14. Medication						
15. Treatment						
16. Management of household						
17. Emotional health						
18. Sleep						
19. Time up during day						
PERFORMANCE SCORE						

Nursing Dependency Index: Professional Sources of Assistance

Patient Code Number ☐☐☐☐   Number of visit ☐☐

	GP	DNS	HV	MSW	ASW	HHS	MOW	VA	CH		DH	OT	PT	Res	Oth	Act. Sc.
Professional Source of Assistance																
1. Bed																
2. Dressing																
3. Walking																
4. Toileting																
5. Provision of meal																
6. Feeding																
7. Control of Environment																
8. Washing and grooming																
9. Bathing or shower																
10. Chair																
11. Wheelchair																
12. Bladder Function																
13. Bowel Function																
14. Medication																
15. Treatment																
16. Management of household																
17. Emotional health																
18. Sleep																
19. Time up during day																
Professional Sources Score																

Nursing Dependency Index: Domestic Sources of Assistance

Patient Code Number ☐☐☐☐   Number of visit ☐☐

Activity	Domestic Sources of Assistance						Activity Score
	Caring Responsible Person*	Other Family Living at home	Other Family Living Away from home	Friends and/or other Relatives	Neigh-bours	Private Domestic Help	
1. Bed							
2. Dressing							
3. Walking							
4. Toileting							
5. Provision of meal							
6. Feeding							
7. Control of Environment							
8. Washing and grooming							
9. Bathing or shower							
10. Chair							
11. Wheelchair							
12. Bladder Function							
13. Bowel Function							
14. Medication							
15. Treatment							
16. Management of household							
17. Emotional health							
18. Sleep							
19. Time up during day							
DOMESTIC SOURCES SCORE							

* Defined as the person accepting moral responsibility for the well being of patient

Nursing Dependency Index
Definitions of Categories of Domestic Sources of Assistance

Please Circle Relevant Definitions for Each Patient – 1 Sheet per Visit		
Caring responsible Person Living with Patient	Other Family living at home	Other Family Living away from home
Husband/Wife Son/Daughter Father/Mother Brother/Sister Aunt/Uncle/Cousin Companion/Friend	Son/Daughter Son/Daughter in law Brother/Sister Brother/Sister in law	Son/Daughter Son/Daughter in law Brother/Sister Brother/Sister in law . . . .

Friends and/or Other Relatives not Living with Patient	Neighbours	Private Domestic Help
As above	Person(s) unrelated to Patient living in neighbourhood	Person employed by Patient for household tasks

Activities of Living Assessment

INTERVIEWER

INTERVIEW NO.
(i.e. 1, 2 or 3)   ☐ 154

Nursing Dependency Score

Total Dependency score   ☐   ☐
                                                155   156

Total dependency requiring human assistance   ☐   ☐
                                                157   158

Domestic sources   ☐   ☐
                                                159   160

Professional sources   ☐   ☐
                                                161   162

Bed   ☐ 163

Dressings   ☐ 164

Mobility   ☐ 165

Hygiene   ☐ 166

Preparation – hot drink, simple snack   ☐ 167

Feeding   ☐ 168

Environment   ☐ 169

Washing and Grooming   ☐ 170

Bathing or shower   ☐ 171

Chair   ☐ 172

Wheelchair   ☐ 173

Bladder Function   ☐ 174

Bowel Function   ☐ 175

Medication ☐ 176

Treatment ☐ 177

Management of household ☐ 178

Emotional health ☐ 179

Sleep ☐ 180

Time up during day ☐ 181

Nursing Dependency
Professional Sources of Assistance

General Practitioner
Units of contact
☐ 182 ☐ 183

District Nurse
Units of contact
☐ 184 ☐ 185

Health Visitor
Units of contact
☐ 186 ☐ 187

Social Worker
Units of contact
☐ 188 ☐ 189

Home Help Services
Units of contact
☐ 190 ☐ 191

Meals on wheels
Units of contact
☐ 192 ☐ 193

Voluntary Agencies (W.V.S., B.R.C., C.S.S., C.H.S.A.)
Units of contact
☐ 194 ☐ 195

Chiropodist
Units of contact
☐ 196 ☐ 197

Day Hospital Support
Units of contact
☐ 198 ☐ 199

Nursing Dependency (Cont.)

Occupational Therapist
Units of contact   ☐   ☐
                                                    200   201

Physiotherapist
Units of contact   ☐   ☐
                                                    202   203

Out-patient follow-up
Units of contact   ☐   ☐
                                                    204   205

Others
Units of contact   ☐   ☐
                                                    206   207

Please state nature of contact

_____

_____   ☐ 208

_____

Life Satisfaction Profile

How often do you do the following activities?
(See list below for possible answers)

1. Reading books, newspapers or magazines .... ☐ 209

2. Taking walks .... ☐ 210

3. Sewing, knitting or crocheting .... ☐ 211

4. Watching TV or listening to the Radio .... ☐ 212

5. Visiting friends or relatives at their home .... ☐ 213

6. Making dinner for friends or relatives .... ☐ 214

7. Attending cinema, theatre or sporting events .... ☐ 215

8. Social games (Chess, Dominoes, Cards, Bingo) .... ☐ 216

9. Fishing, hunting, golf, bowling or other sports .... ☐ 217

10. Playing a musical instrument .... ☐ 218

11. Hobbies (Stamp collecting, model making, dressmaking etc) ...... ☐ 219

	Code		*Code*		*Code*
EVERY DAY	6	ONCE A WEEK	4	ONCE A MONTH	2
2 OR 3 TIMES		ABOUT TWICE		A COUPLE OF	
A WEEK	5	A MONTH	3	TIMES A YEAR	1
				NEVER	0
				NO INFORMATION	X

12. Do you belong to any clubs or organisations
    which hold regular meetings?

YES	
NO	
NO INFO.	

☐ 220

13. What are these organisations, and how often
    do they meet? (SEE LIST)

14. How often did you attend meetings? (see list)

....

15. Were you an officer or have any special responsibilities such as chairman or member of a committee? (see list)

....

16. About how much time all together (per week or per month) did you devote to your organisation, including all meetings, functions and other work done?

....

List

Organisation	Frequency of meetings	Time spent	How often patient attended	Positions held and duties

☐ 221
☐ 222
☐ 223
☐ 224

1	2	3
Agree	Disagree	Undecided

Check boxes from right to left within a diagonal line with an X score one point.

17. As I grow older, things seem better than I thought they would be.　　| 1 | 2 | 3 |　　☐ 225

18. I have had more chances in life than most of the people I know.　　| 1 | 2 | 3 |　　☐ 226

19. This is the dreariest time of my life.　　| 1 | 2 | 3 |　　☐ 227

20. I am just as happy now as when I was younger.　　| 1 | 2 | 3 |　　☐ 228

21. My life could be happier than it is now.　　| 1 | 2 | 3 |　　☐ 229

22. These are the best years of my life.　　| 1 | 2 | 3 |　　☐ 230

23. Most of the things I do are boring or monotonous.　　| 1 | 2 | 3 |　　☐ 231

24. I expect some interesting and pleasant things to happen to me in the future.   [1 | 2 | 3]   □ 232

25. The things I do today are as interesting to me as they ever were.   [1 | 2 | 3]   □ 233

26. I feel old and somewhat tired.   [1 | 2 | 3]   □ 234

27. As I look back on my life I am fairly well satisfied.   [1 | 2 | 3]   □ 235

28. I would not change my past even if I could.   [1 | 2 | 3]   □ 236

29. I like to take an interest in my appearance.   [1 | 2 | 3]   □ 237

30. I have made plans for things I'll be doing in a month or a year from now.   [1 | 2 | 3]   □ 238

31. When I think back over my life, I didn't get most of the important things I wanted.   [1 | 2 | 3]   □ 239

32. Compared to other people, I get down in the dumps too often.   [1 | 2 | 3]   □ 240

33. I've got pretty much what I expected out of life.   [1 | 2 | 3]   □ 241

34. In spite of what people say, the life of the average person is getting worse not better.   [1 | 2 | 3]   □ 242

Total Score LSi – A   Boxes with an X score one point.   □   □
                                                             243   244

1. While you were in hospital were you given any advice about what you should or should not do during your convalescence?

   Yes = 1 No = 2   ☐ 245

2. If yes, please say what:

   _____   246☐☐247
   _____   248   249
   _____   250☐☐251
   _____   252   253

3. Would you have liked more information or advice?   254☐☐255
   Yes = 1 No = 2   ☐ 256

4. If yes, please specify: 257☐☐258
                                                          259   260
   _____   261☐☐262
                                                          263   264
   _____   265☐☐266

5. What was good about the nursing you received in hospital?   267☐☐268
                                                          269   270
   _____   271☐☐272

   _____

6. What was not so good about the nursing you received in hospital?
   _____   273☐☐274
                                                          275   276
   _____   277☐☐278

7. Here is a lot of unfinished sentences, would you try and complete these for me?

   (a) The most difficult thing to ask the nurse about was

   _____   ☐ 279
   (b) As far as the nurses were concerned, I always knew

   _____   ☐ 280
   (c) The nurses always

   _____   ☐ 281
   (d) If it hadn't been for the nurses, I would have

   _____   ☐ 282
   (e) Before going home, I would have liked it if

   _____   ☐ 283

8.   Frankly I would like to know what problems you have had since   284☐☐285
      discharge, and if you have been able to cope with them.   286   287
                                                                            288☐☐289
                                                                            290   291
                                                                            292☐☐293

9.   Have you returned to work?   Yes = 1 No = 2
                                                          Not applicable = 3   ☐ 294

10.   If 9 = Yes, number of days post-op you started work.   295☐☐296

Nursing Dependency Index

Patient Code Number ☐☐☐☐   Date of Visit ☐☐☐☐☐☐   Number of Visit ☐☐

Day Base ....   Interval since last visit (in days) ☐☐

Activity* Important note: Only score ONE performance per activity						
*See Definition Sheet Performance of A.D.L. activity	Independent	Independent with aids	Required Assistance of no more than 1 person	Requires Assistance of no more than 2 persons	Bedfast	Activity Score
1. Bed	Score 1 /activity	Score 2 /activity	Score 3 /activity	Score 4 /activity	Score 5 /activity	
2. Dressing						
3. Walking						
4. Toileting						
5. Provision of meal						
6. Feeding						
7. Control of environment						
8. Washing and grooming						
9. Bathing or shower						
10. Chair						
11. Wheelchair						
12. Bladder function						
13. Bowel function						
14. Medication						
15. Treatment						
16. Management of household						
17. Emotional health						
18. Sleep						
19. Time up during day						
PERFORMANCE SCORE						

Nursing Dependency Index: Professional Sources of Assistance

Patient Code Number ▢▢▢▢   Number of visit ▢▢

Professional Source of Assistance															
	GP	DNS	HV	MSW	ASW	HHS	MOW	VA	CH		DH	OT	PT	Res	Oth	Act. Sc.
1. Bed																
2. Dressing																
3. Walking																
4. Toileting																
5. Provision of meal																
6. Feeding																
7. Control of Environment																
8. Washing and grooming																
9. Bathing or shower																
10. Chair																
11. Wheelchair																
12. Bladder Function																
13. Bowel Function																
14. Medication																
15. Treatment																
16. Management of household																
17. Emotional health																
18. Sleep																
19. Time up during day																
Professional Sources Score																

Nursing Dependency Index: Domestic Sources of Assistance

Patient Code Number ☐☐☐☐   Number of visit ☐☐

Activity	Domestic Sources of Assistance						Activity Score
	Caring Responsible Person*	Other Family Living at home	Other Family Living Away from home	Friends and/or other Relatives	Neigh-bours	Private Domestic Help	
1. Bed							
2. Dressing							
3. Walking							
4. Toileting							
5. Provision of meal							
6. Feeding							
7. Control of Environment							
8. Washing and grooming							
9. Bathing or shower							
10. Chair							
11. Wheelchair							
12. Bladder Function							
13. Bowel Function							
14. Medication							
15. Treatment							
16. Management of household							
17. Emotional health							
18. Sleep							
19. Time up during day							
DOMESTIC SOURCES SCORE							

* Defined as the person accepting moral responsibility for the well being of patient

Nursing Dependency Index
Definitions of Categories of Domestic Sources of Assistance

Please Circle Relevant Definitions for Each Patient – 1 Sheet per Visit		
Caring responsible Person Living with Patient	Other Family living at home	Other Family Living away from home
Husband/Wife Son/Daughter Father/Mother Brother/Sister Aunt/Uncle/Cousin Companion/Friend	Son/Daughter Son/Daughter in law Brother/Sister Brother/Sister in law	Son/Daughter Son/Daughter in law Brother/Sister Brother/Sister in law ....

Friends and/or Other Relatives not Living with Patient	Neighbours	Private Domestic Help
As above	Person(s) unrelated to Patient living in neighbourhood	Person employed by Patient for household tasks

Activities of Living Assessment

INTERVIEWER

INTERVIEW NO.
(i.e. 1, 2 or 3)   ☐ 297

Nursing Dependency Score

Total Dependency score   ☐   ☐
                                                          298   299

Total dependency requiring human assistance   ☐   ☐
                                                          300   301

Domestic sources   ☐   ☐
                                                          302   303

Professional sources   ☐   ☐
                                                          304   305

Bed   ☐ 306

Dressings   ☐ 307

Mobility   ☐ 308

Hygiene   ☐ 309

Preparation – hot drink, simple snack   ☐ 310

Feeding   ☐ 311

Environment   ☐ 312

Washing and Grooming   ☐ 313

Bathing or shower   ☐ 314

Chair   ☐ 315

Wheelchair   ☐ 316

Bladder Function   ☐ 317

Bowel Function   ☐ 318

Medication	☐ 319
Treatment	☐ 320
Management of household	☐ 321
Emotional health	☐ 322
Sleep	☐ 323
Time up during day	☐ 324

Nursing Dependency
Professional Sources of Assistance

General Practitioner
Units of contact   ☐ 325   ☐ 326

District Nurse
Units of contact   ☐ 327   ☐ 328

Health Visitor
Units of contact   ☐ 329   ☐ 330

Social Worker
Units of contact   ☐ 331   ☐ 332

Home Help Services
Units of contact   ☐ 333   ☐ 334

Meals on wheels
Units of contact   ☐ 335   ☐ 336

Voluntary Agencies (W.V.S., B.R.C., C.S.S., C.H.S.A.)
Units of contact   ☐ 337   ☐ 338

Chiropodist
Units of contact   ☐ 339   ☐ 340

Day Hospital Support
Units of contact   ☐ 341   ☐ 342

Nursing Dependency (Cont.)

Occupational Therapist

Units of contact

☐   ☐
343   344

Physiotherapist

Units of contact

☐   ☐
345   346

Out-patient follow-up

Units of contact

☐   ☐
347   348

Others

Units of contact

☐   ☐
349   350

Please state nature of contact

_____

_____   ☐ 351

_____

Life Satisfaction Profile

How often do you do the following activities?
(See list below for possible answers)

1. Reading books, newspapers or magazines .... ☐ 352

2. Taking walks .... ☐ 353

3. Sewing, knitting or crocheting .... ☐ 354

4. Watching TV or listening to the Radio .... ☐ 355

5. Visiting friends or relatives at their home .... ☐ 356

6 Making dinner for friends or relatives .... ☐ 357

7. Attending cinema, theatre or sporting events .... ☐ 358

8. Social games (Chess, Dominoes, Cards, Bingo) .... ☐ 359

9. Fishing, hunting, golf, bowling or other sports .... ☐ 360

10. Playing a musical instrument .... ☐ 361

11. Hobbies (Stamp collecting, model making, dressmaking etc) ...... ☐ 362

	Code		*Code*		*Code*
EVERY DAY	6	ONCE A WEEK	4	ONCE A MONTH	2
2 OR 3 TIMES		ABOUT TWICE		A COUPLE OF	
A WEEK	5	A MONTH	3	TIMES A YEAR	1
				NEVER	0
				NO INFORMATION	X

12. Do you belong to any clubs or organisations which hold regular meetings?

YES	
NO	
NO INFO.	

☐ 363

13. What are these organisations, and how often do they meet? (SEE LIST)

14. How often did you attend meetings? (see list)
. . . .

15. Were you an officer or have any special responsibilities such as chairman or member of a committee? (see list)
. . . .

16. About how much time all together (per week or per month) did you devote to your organisation, including all meetings, functions and other work done?
. . . .

List

Organisation	Frequency of meetings	Time spent	How often patient attended	Positions held and duties

☐ 364
☐ 365
☐ 366
☐ 367

1	2	3
Agree	Disagree	Undecided

Check boxes from right to left within a diagonal line with an X score one point.

17. As I grow older, things seem better than I thought they would be. `1 2 3`   ☐ 368

18. I have had more chances in life than most of the people I know. `1 2 3`   ☐ 369

19. This is the dreariest time of my life. `1 2 3`   ☐ 370

20. I am just as happy now as when I was younger. `1 2 3`   ☐ 371

21. My life could be happier than it is now. `1 2 3`   ☐ 372

22. These are the best years of my life. `1 2 3`   ☐ 373

23. Most of the things I do are boring or monotonous. `1 2 3`   ☐ 374

24. I expect some interesting and pleasant things to happen to me in the future. | 1 | 2 | 3 | ☐ 375

25. The things I do today are as interesting to me as they ever were. | 1 | 2 | 3 | ☐ 376

26. I feel old and somewhat tired. | 1 | 2 | 3 | ☐ 377

27. As I look back on my life I am fairly well satisfied. | 1 | 2 | 3 | ☐ 378

28. I would not change my past even if I could. | 1 | 2 | 3 | ☐ 379

29. I like to take an interest in my appearance | 1 | 2 | 3 | ☐ 380

30. I have made plans for things I'll be doing in a month or a year from now. | 1 | 2 | 3 | ☐ 381

31. When I think back over my life, I didn't get most of the important things I wanted. | 1 | 2 | 3 | ☐ 382

32. Compared to other people, I get down in the dumps too often. | 1 | 2 | 3 | ☐ 383

33. I've got pretty much what I expected out of life. | 1 | 2 | 3 | ☐ 384

34. In spite of what people say, the life of the average person is getting worse not better. | 1 | 2 | 3 | ☐ 385

Total Score LSI – A Boxes with an X score one point. ☐ 386 ☐ 387

35. I would like to know what problems you have had since the last two interviews and if you have been able to cope with them. 388☐☐389 390☐☐391 392☐☐393
_____
_____

36. Have you returned to work yet? Yes=1 No=2 ☐ 394

37. If 36=Yes, number of days post op on day work started ☐☐☐ 395 396 397

References

Alfano G J (1969) A professional approach to nursing practice. *Nursing Clinics of North America,* **4**(3): 487–493.

Alfano G J (1971) Healing or caretaking – which will it be? *Nursing Clinics of North America,* **6**: 273–280.

Ahlsiö B, Britton M, Murray V and Theorell T (1984) Disablement and quality of life after stroke. *Stroke,* **15**(5): 886–890.

Batchelor I (1980) The multidisciplinary clinical team – a working paper. London: Kings Fund.

Boore J (1978) *A Prescription for Recovery.* London: Royal College of Nursing.

Bower F L (1972) *The Process of Planning Nursing Care.* St Louis: C V Mosby.

Bower F L (1977) The process of planning nursing care: a theoretical model. *Kango Gijutsu,* **23**: 143–147.

Bukowski L, Bonavolonta M, Keehn M T and Morgan K A (1986) Interdisciplinary roles in stroke care. *Nursing Clinics of North America,* **21**(2): 359–374.

Byrne M L and Thompson L F (1978) *Key Concepts for the Study and Practice of Nursing,* 2nd edn. St Louis: C V Mosby.

Capra F (1982) *The Turning Point: Science, Society and the Rising Culture.* London: Fontana.

Chapman C (1979) Sociological theory related to nursing. In: Colledge M M and Jones D (eds), *Readings in Nursing.* Edinburgh: Churchill Livingstone.

Clay T (1987) *Nurses: Power and Politics.* London: Heinemann Medical Books.

Daeffler R J (1975) Patients' perception of care under team and primary nursing. *Journal of Nursing Administration,* **5**(3): 20–26.

Davis B (1984) Preoperative information giving: an implementation study, report to SHHD, NRU Edinburgh, core program project.

DeJong G and Branch L G (1982) Predicting the stroke patient's ability to live independently. *Stroke,* **13**(5): 648–655.

Department of Health and Social Security (1980) *Nursing Homes: Their Role in the Care of Elderly People.* London: HMSO.

Egan G (1975) *The Skilled Helper.* California: Brooks/Cole, Monterey.

Egger J and Stix P (1984) The coping process with illness in patients with cardiovascular or cerebrovascular diseases: a new survey: EKV. *International Journal of Rehabilitation Research.* **7**(2).

Field D (1972) Disability as social deviance. In: *Medical Men and Their Work.* (Friedson, E, Corber, J, eds). New York: Aldine Atherton.

Friedson E (1970) *Professional Dominance. The Social Structure of Health Care.* Chicago: Adine.

Friedson E (1975) *The Profession of Medicine.* New York: Dodds, Mead & Co.

Garroway, W M, Akhtar A J, Prescott R J and Hockey L (1980) Management of acute stroke in the elderly: preliminary results of a controlled trial. *British Medical Journal,* **280:** 1040–1043.

Gonzalez F (1981) How should nursing be managed below the level of director of nursing services? *Nursing Times.* **77**(14): 604–605.

Graham H and Livesey B (1983) Can readmissions to a geriatric medical unit be prevented? *The Lancet,* 19 February.

Hall L E (1964) Project report, the Solomon and Betty Loeb Centre for Nursing, Montefiore Hospital, The Centre, New York.

Hall L E (1966) Another view of nursing care and quality. In: Straub M and Parker K (eds), *Continuity of Patient Care: The Role of Nursing.* Washington DC: Catholic University of America Press.

Hall L E (1969) The Loeb Centre for Nursing and Rehabilitation, Montefiore Hospital and Medical Centre, Bronx, New York, *International Journal of Nursing Studies,* **6:** 81–95.

Hall L, Alfons G, Rifkin E and Levine H (1975) Final report: longitudinal effects of an experimental nursing process unpublished, New York, Loeb Centre for Nursing Project report, the Solomon and Betty Loeb Centre, Montefiore Hospital, The Centre, New York.

Hawthorn P (1974) *Nurse I Want My Mummy.* London: Royal College of Nursing.

Hayward J (1975) *Information – A Prescription Against Pain.* London: Royal College of Nursing.

Hegyvary S T and Haussman R K D (1976) Monitoring nursing care quality. *Journal of Nursing Administration,* **6:** 9.

Helt E H and Pelikan J A (1975) Quality: medical care's answer to Madison Avenue. *American Journal of Public Health,* **65:** 284–290.

Henderson V (1966) *The Nature of Nursing.* London: Collier Macmillan.

Herman J M, Culpepper L and Franks P (1984) Patterns of utilization, disposition, and length of stay among stroke patients in a community hospital setting. *Journal of the American Geriatric Society,* **32**(6): 421–426.

Hockey L (1985) *Nursing Research: Mistakes and Misconceptions.* Edinburgh: Churchill Livingstone.

Johnson M M and Davis M L C (1975) *Problem Solving in Nursing Practice.* Iowa: Wm C Brown Co.

Jourard S (1971) *The Transparent Self.* New York: D Van Nostrand.

Katz S and Akpom C A (1976) A measure of primary sociobiological functions. *International Journal of Health Services,* **6:** 3.

Kitson A (1984) Steps toward the identification and development of nursing therapeutic functions in the care of hospitalized elderly, unpublished PhD thesis, University of Ulster, Coleraine.

Kreiger D (1981) *Foundations for Holistic Health Practices.* Philadelphia: J. B. Lippincott Co.

La Monica E (1979) *The Nursing Process — A Humanistic Approach.* California: Addison Wesley.

Lawrence L and Christie D (1979) Quality of life after stroke: a three year follow-up. *Age and ageing,* **8**(3): 167–172.

Lehmann J F, DeLateur B J, Fowler R S, Warren C G, Arnhold R, Scheatzer G, Hurka R, Whitmore J J, Masock A J and Chamber K H. (1975) Stroke: does rehabilitation affect outcome? Stroke rehabilitation: outcome and prediction. *Archives of Physical Medicine,* **56**(9): 375–389.

Lind K (1982) A synthesis of studies on stroke rehabilitation. *Journal of Chronic Diseases,* **35**: part 2.

McFarlane J K (1976) The role of research and the development of nursing theory. *Journal of Advanced Nursing,* **1**: 443–451.

McMahon R A (1986) Nursing as a therapy. *The Professional Nurse,* July, 270–272.

Manthey M (1980) *The Practice of Primary Nursing,* Oxford: Blackwell Scientific Publications.

Manthey M and Kramer M S (1970) A dialogue on primary nursing. *Nursing Forum,* **9**: 356–379.

Marram G, Schlegal M and Bevis E (1974) *Primary Nursing.* St Louis: C V Mosby.

Mechanic D (1975) Ideology, medical technology, and health care organisations in modern nations. *American Journal of Public Health,* **65**: 241–247.

Neugarten B L, Havighirst R J and Tobin S S (1961) The measurement of life satisfaction. *Journal of Gerontology,* **16**: 134–143.

Neuman B (1980) The Betty Neuman health care systems model: a total person approach to patient problems. In: Riehl J P and Roy C (eds), *Conceptual Models for Nursing Practice.* New York: Appleton Century Crofts.

Norton D, McClaren R and Exton-Smith A M (1962) *An Investigation of Geriatric Nursing Problems in Hospitals* (reprinted 1975). Edinburgh: Churchill Livingstone.

Orem D E (1966) Discussion of paper by L E Hall: 'Another view of nursing care equality'. In: Straub M and Parker K (eds), *Continuity of Patient Care; the role of Nursing.* Washington DC: Catholic University of America Press.

Orem D E (1980) *Nursing: Concepts of Practice.* New York: McGraw Hill.

Parsons T (1951) *The Social System.* London: Routledge and Kegan Paul.

Pearson A (1983) *The Clinical Nursing Unit.* London: Heineman Medical.

Pearson A (1985) The effects of introducing new norms into a nursing unit and an analysis of the process of change, unpublished PhD thesis, Department of Social Science, University of London, Goldsmiths College.

Pearson A (ed.) (1987a) *Nursing Quality Measurement – Quality Assurance Methods for Peer Review.* Chicester: John Wiley.

Pearson A (ed.) (1987b) *Primary Nursing: Nursing in the Burford Oxford Nursing Development Units.* London: Croom Helm.

Pearson A, Smith A, Punton S and Durand I (1987) Nursing beds – an alternative health care provision, unpublished report, Oxford.

Pearson A and Vaughan B A (1986) *Nursing Models for Practice.* London: Heineman.

Pearson A and Vaughan B (1984) Module 1: Nursing practice and the nursing process. In: *A Systematic Approach to Nursing Care – an Introduction.* Milton Keynes: Open University.

Pembury S (1984) In praise of competence. *Lampada,* **1:** 12.

Poirer B (1975) Loeb Centre: what nursing can and should be. *The American Nurse,* **7:** 5.

Reilly D (1975) Why a conceptual framework? *Nursing Outlook,* **23:** 9.

Riehl J P and Roy C (1980) *Conceptual Models for Nursing Practice.* New York: Appleton Century Crofts.

Roper N (1976) *Clinical Experience in Nursing Education.* Edinburgh: Churchill Livingstone.

Roper N (1979) Nursing based on a model of living. In: Colledge M M and Jones D (eds), *Readings in Nursing.* Edinburgh: Churchill Livingstone.

Roper N, Logan W W and Tierney A J (1980) *The Elements of Nursing.* Edinburgh: Churchill Livingstone.

Roper N, Logan W W and Tierney A J (1981) *Learning to Use the Process of Nursing.* Edinburgh: Churchill Livingstone.

Roper N, Logan W W and Tierney A J (1983) *Using a Model for Nursing.* Edinburgh: Churchill Livingstone.

Rottkamp B C (1985) A holistic approach to identifying factors associated with an altered pattern of urinary elimination in stroke patients. *The American Association of Neuroscience Nurses.* **17**(1): 37–44.

Roy C (1980) The Roy adaptation model. In: Riehl J P and Roy C (eds). *Conceptual Models for Nursing Practice.* New York: Appleton Century Crofts.

Saxton D F and Hyland P A (1975) *Planning and Implementing Nursing Intervention.* St Louis: C V Mosby.

Schaffrath W B (1978) Commission leads way to joint practice for nurses and physicians. *Hospitals,* **52:** 78–81.

Sjögren K (1982) Leisure after stroke. *International Rehabilitation Medicine,* **4:** 2.

Smuts J C (1926) *Holism and Evolution.* New York: Macmillan.

Sparrow S (1986) Primary Nursing. *Nursing Practitioner,* **1**(3): 142–148.

Stannard C (1973) Old folks and dirty work: the social conditions for patient abuse in a nursing home. *Social Problems,* **20:** 329–342.

Stockwell F (1972) *The Unpopular Patient.* London: Royal College of Nursing.

Sundeen S J, Stuart G W, Rankin E D and Cohen S P (1976) *Nurse-Client Interaction – Implementing the Nursing Process.* St Louis: C V Mosby.

Swaffield L (1983) A model for the future? *Nursing Times,* 12 January, 13–16.

Tiffany C H (1977) Nursing, organizational structure and the real goals of hospitals: a correlational study, unpublished PhD study, Indiana University.

Towell D (1975) *Understanding Psychiatric Nursing.* London: Royal College of Nursing.

Travelbee J (1971) *Interpersonal Aspects of Nursing.* Philadelphia: F A Davies and Co.

Tutton L (1987) My very own nurse. *Nursing Times,* **83**(38): 27–29.

Wilson-Barnett J (1984) *Key Functions in Nursing.* London: Royal College of Nursing.

Wright S G (1986) Nursing as a therapy. *The Professional Nurse,* July, 270–272.

Yura H and Walsh M B (1973) *The Nursing Process.* New York: Appleton Century Crofts.